Multiple Choice Questions in Pediatric Dentistry

Multiple Choice Questions in Pediatric Dentistry

Dr. M. S. Muthu, MDS
Associate Professor
Department of Pedodontics
Meenakshi Ammal Dental College
Maduravoyil, Chennai (India)

ELSEVIER

ELSEVIER
A division of
Reed Elsevier India Pvt. Ltd.

Multiple Choice Questions in Pediatric Dentistry
Muthu

ELSEVIER
A division of
Reed Elsevier India Private Limited

Mosby, Saunders, Churchill Livingstone, Butterworth Heinemann and Hanley & Belfus are the Health Science imprints of Elsevier.

First Edition 2005

ISBN-13: 978-81-8147-855-9
ISBN-10: 81-8147-855-X

Published by Elsevier, a division of Reed Elsevier India Private Limited, 17-A/1, Main Ring Road, Lajpat Nagar - IV, New Delhi-110 024 (India).

Typeset at DataVision, D-2, MCD Flat, R-Block GK-I, ND-48.

Printed and bound at Rajkamal Electric Press, Delhi.

To
my beloved parents
Mr. Murugan and Mrs. Balasaraswathi
and
my loving wife Prathibha

Foreword

I am delighted to introduce this book written by Dr. M.S. Muthu on Multiple Choice Questions in Pediatric Dentistry.

It is really heartening to know that one of my students has put in tremendous hard work to bring out this book for the benefit of students of dentistry.

Dr. Muthu had excelled in pediatric dental practice; both as clinician and academician. Very few books on MCQs in Pediatric Dentistry are available. This book fills the gap. The questions are meticulously selected by the author, which needs appreciation.

I am sure this book will be accepted by undergraduate students as it would encourage them to detect the areas of weakness in their understanding of the subject so that they may return to the text for a more comprehensive review of the topics. Also this book will serve the need and prove extremely useful for students in preparing themselves for competitive exams.

The author deserves to be congratulated for an excellent, well co-ordinated academic venture.

Prof. S.G. Damle
Prof. & Head
Dept. of Pediatric Dentistry &
Dean, Nair Hospital Dental College
Mumbai

Preface

This is an elaborate and penetrating collection of multiple choice questions in the subject of Pediatric Dentistry. This project was primarily taken up by me with the aim of helping the undergraduate and post-graduate students of dentistry to strengthen their basics in this upcoming field.

The competitive examinations of these days demand a sound knowledge of the fundamentals of any subject. Preparation for these entrance exams does not end with merely reading the textbooks. It becomes complete only when the concepts are repeatedly revised by solving the related multiple choice questions.

In this book I have presented about 800 multiple choice questions with relevant explanations. They are organized in a chapterwise manner for the convenience of students. All the questions were framed with the idea of emphasizing the important facts and points pertaining to each chapter. I have provided clear explanations for most of the questions along with relevant tables, related information and images, which will definitely help the students to understand the subject better.

I would sincerely urge the students to repeatedly revise these questions along with their explanations in order to make the most out of this book.

I am sure this book will serve its prime purpose of helping the students to master the fundamentals of Pediatric dentistry.

M. S. Muthu

Acknowledgements

My heartfelt thanks to:

My teachers and mentors who have shaped me into what I am.

My students who have inspired me to write this book.

Dr. E. Munirathinam Naidu, an inspiring teacher who has provided the most conducive environment for me to work.

Dr. N. Sivakumar, for his valuable comments and constant encouragement.

My postgraduate students (especially Dr. Sarath Asokan, Dr. EMG Subramanian), junior doctors (Dr. Shifa, Dr. Nirmal and Dr. Soundar) for helping me to proof read and complete this manuscript.

Ms. Jeyashree, for helping me proof read this manuscript.

Ms. Sam, an excellent photographer who has captured the images for me.

My parent, my father in law, Ganesh, Anu, Srini, Vasanthi and Gayatri for their support and encouragement in all my endeavours.

My wife, for giving me all her time and love to make this work complete.

M. S. Muthu

Contents

Chapter 1

Diagnosis and Treatment Planning

1. Based on the universal system of dental recording (Tooth Charting System) the number given for left maxillary first permanent molar is:

(*a*) 1 (*b*) 6

(*c*) 14 (*d*) 16

Answer (*c*).

In the universal system, the marking of permanent teeth is done with the numbers 1 to 32 beginning with the upper right third molar (No. 1) progressing around the arch to the upper left third molar (No. 16), down to the lower left third molar (No. 17) and around the arch to the lower right third molar (No. 32). The primary teeth are identified in the universal system by the first 20 letters of the alphabets (from A to T). Upper right second primary molar is denoted as A thereafter progressing around the arch to the upper left second primary molar (J), down to the lower left second primary molar (K) and around the arch to the lower right second primary molar (T).

1	2	3	4	5	6	7	8	9	10	11	12	13	14	15	16
32	31	30	29	28	27	26	25	24	23	22	21	20	19	18	17

ABCDE	FGHIJ
TSRQP	ONMLK

Hence 14 denotes maxillary left first permanent molar. Maxillary right third molar is denoted by the number 1. Maxillary right canine and maxillary left third molar are denoted by 6 and 16, respectively.

2. According to the universal system, the 20 primary teeth are identified by the letters of the alphabet as follows:

(*a*) A to T (*b*) A to E

(*c*) A to J (*d*) a to e

Answer (*a*).

Alphabets A to T denote the 20 primary teeth whereas alphabets a to e are not used in the universal system to denote the primary teeth.

3. In the FDI system of dental recording, which of the following is true?

(*a*) The first digit indicates the quadrant and the second digit the type of tooth within the quadrant.

(*b*) Quadrants are allotted the digits 1 to 4 for the permanent teeth and 5 to 8 for the primary teeth in a clockwise sequence, starting from the upper right side.

(*c*) Teeth within the same quadrant are allotted the digits 1 to 8 (primary teeth 1 to 5) from the midline backwards.

(*d*) This is known as the two-digit system and the digits should be pronounced separately.

(*e*) All of the above.

Answer (*e*).

All the above mentioned facts are correct.

18 17 16 15 14 13 12 11	21 22 23 24 25 26 27 28
48 47 46 45 44 43 42 41	31 32 33 34 35 36 37 38
55 54 53 52 51	61 62 63 64 65
85 84 83 82 81	71 72 73 74 75

4. The carious lesion always appears smaller on the radiograph than it actually is. Likewise, microscopic observation of ground sections of teeth reveals that progress of the lesion through the enamel and dentin is more extensive than is evident on the radiograph.

(*a*) Both the statements are false.

(*b*) Both the statements are true.

(*c*) First statement is true and the second is false.

(*d*) First statement is false and the second is true.

Answer (*b*).

The answer is self-explanatory.

5. The child's first dental visit and oral examinations should take place by at least:

(*a*) 1 year of age

(*b*) 3 years of age

(*c*) 6 years of age

(*d*) 4 years of age

Answer (*a*).

The child's first dental visit and oral examination should take place by at least one year of age or as soon as the primary teeth start erupting. This early dental visit helps the dentist and the parents to discuss ways to nurture excellent oral health before any serious problem develops. Previously it was considered (apt) to start the first dental visit by three years of age because by then the child would have grown enough to cooperate with the dentist for examination.

6. Which of the following is true about performing an infant examination?

(*a*) Done in knee to knee position.

(*b*) Done in an area with adequate light for visual examination.

(*c*) An assistant required to help hold the child's attention so that parents can concentrate on the information being given.

(*d*) All of the above.

Answer (*d*).

All the above mentioned factors are true with regard to infant examination.

7. Which of the following is true regarding drug abuse?

(*a*) Symptoms of abuse may include depression, frustration, feeling of inadequacy, helplessness, immaturity, major deficiencies in ego structure and functioning.

(*b*) Substances commonly abused are solvents, inhalants, narcotics stimulants, sedatives, tranquilizers and tobacco.

(*c*) Glue sniffing and gasoline sniffing are also different forms of drug abuse.

(*d*) All of the above.

Answer (*d*).

All the above mentioned factors are true regarding substance abuse.

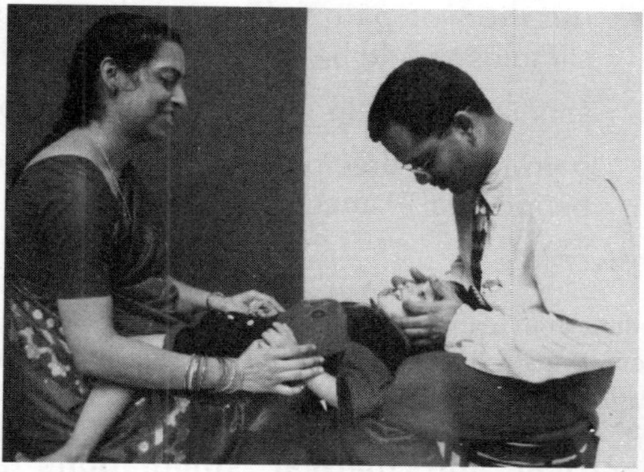

Fig. 1.1 Infant examination.

8. In extra oral assessment the height and weight information is recorded for:

(*a*) correlating it with dental disease

(*b*) establishing the relationship with early childhood caries

(*c*) comparing with the standard growth curves

(*d*) none of the above

Answer (*c*).

The height and weight information is recorded to compare them with the standard growth curves. If a patient is below the 3rd percentile or above the 97th percentile referral to a pediatrician becomes necessary.

9. All of the following statements are true regarding pain history taking except:

(*a*) child should be asked whether hot or cold food or drinks have any relation to pain.

(*b*) duration of pain following the exposure to stimulus should be questioned.

(*c*) spontaneous pain indicates reversible pulpitis.

(*d*) pain that is precipitated by pressure indicates periodontal damage.

Answer (*c*).

Spontaneous pain indicates irreversible pulpitis. Eliciting an accurate pain history can be very useful in determining the treatment planning for child.

10. Electrical and thermal stimulations are the most common methods of assessing vitality. Young children are not good candidates for vitality testing as false positive responses are common in primary dentition.

(*a*) Both the statements are true.

(*b*) Both the statements are false.

(*c*) First statement is true and the second is false.

(*d*) First statement is false and the second is true.

Answers (*a*).

The answer is self-explanatory.

11. In caries risk assessment which of the following factors are evaluated?

(*a*) Medical and social history

(*b*) Dietary habits

(*c*) Fluoride use

(*d*) Plaque control

(*e*) All of the above

Answer (*e*).

The answer is self-explanatory. Past caries experience is also recorded as part of the caries risk assessment protocol.

Chapter 2

Morphology and Development of Primary and Permanent Teeth

1. Evidence of development of human tooth can be observed as early as:

(*a*) 6th week of embryonic life

(*b*) 11th week of embryonic life

(*c*) 14th week of embryonic life

(*d*) 16th week of embryonic life

Answer (*a*).

Evidence of development of tooth can be observed as early as 6th week of embryonic life. According to Kraus and Jordan the first macroscopic indication of morphologic development of tooth occurs at approximately 11 weeks in utero. Calcification of the primary maxillary central incisor begins at approximately 14 weeks in utero. Evidence of developing primary canines can be observed between 14–16 weeks.

2. Microdontia or macrodontia of teeth is because of damage in __________ stage of tooth development:

(*a*) initiation/proliferation

(*b*) histodifferentiation

(*c*) morphodifferentiation

(*d*) apposition

Answer (*c*).

Microdontia or macrodontia of teeth is because of damage occurring in the stage of morphodifferentiation.

S.No.	***Aberration in stage of tooth development***	***Result***
1.	Initiation/ Proliferation	Supernumerary teeth Partial anodontia Odontoma
2.	Histodifferentiation	Amelogenesis imperfecta Dentinogenesis imperfecta
3.	Morphodifferentiation	Peg teeth Mulberry molars Microdontia Macrodontia Talon cusp
4.	Apposition	Enamel hypoplasia Interglobular dentin

3. Enamel hypoplasia is because of disturbance in __________ stage of tooth development:

(*a*) initiation/proliferation

(*b*) histodifferentiation

(*c*) morphodifferentiation

(*d*) apposition

Answer (*d*).

Refer to the explanation of Q. No. 2.

4. The first macroscopic indication of morphologic development of primary incisors occurs approximately at:

(*a*) 11 weeks in utero (*b*) 14 weeks in utero

(*c*) 16 weeks in utero (*d*) 6 weeks in utero

Answer (*a*).

Kraus and Jordan have found that the first macroscopic indication of morphologic development occurs at approximately 11 weeks in utero. The maxillary and mandibular central incisor crowns appear identical at this early stage as tiny, hemispheric, mound like structures.

5. The first evidence of calcification of primary teeth begins approximately at:

(*a*) 11 weeks in utero (*b*) 14 weeks in utero

(*c*) 16 weeks in utero (*d*) 6 weeks in utero

Answer (*b*).

Calcification of the primary maxillary central incisor begins at approximately 14 weeks in utero, the upper central incisor slightly preceding the lower central.

6. In primary teeth, cusp of Carabelli is seen in:

(*a*) maxillary first molar

(*b*) maxillary second molar
(*c*) mandibular first molar
(*d*) mandibular second molar

Answer (*b*).

Cusp of Carabelli is seen in maxillary second primary molar. Mandibular first primary molar has a central ridge.

7. The primary tooth which least resembles any of the permanent tooth is:

(*a*) maxillary first molar
(*b*) maxillary second molar
(*c*) mandibular first molar
(*d*) mandibular second molar

Answer (*c*).

Mandibular first molar is the tooth which least resembles any permanent tooth. It has a prominent buccal curvature. Maxillary second primary molar resembles the maxillary first permanent molar. Mandibular second primary molar resembles the mandibular second permanent molar.

8. Extreme curvature of the buccal side is characteristic of:

(*a*) mandibular first primary molar
(*b*) mandibular second primary molar
(*c*) maxillary first molar
(*d*) maxillary second primary molar

Answer (*a*).

Extreme curvature of the buccal side is characteristic of mandibular first primary molar. The buccal curvature of maxillary first primary molar is not as prominent as the mandibular first primary molar.

9. The primary second molar (mandibular) resembles:

(*a*) maxillary first permanent molar

(*b*) mandibular first permanent molar

(*c*) maxillary second permanent molar

(*d*) mandibular second permanent molar

Answer (*b*).

Mandibular second primary molar resembles the mandibular first permanent molar. Maxillary second primary molar resembles the maxillary first permanent molar. Maxillary and mandibular second permanent molar do not resemble any primary tooth.

10. All of the following are true of primary teeth except:

(*a*) crowns of the primary tooth are wider in comparison to their crown length than are permanent teeth

(*b*) roots of primary molars are long and slender

(*c*) primary teeth are usually lighter in colour than the permanent teeth

(*d*) buccal curvature on primary first molars are not prominent

Answer (*d*).

Extreme curvature of the buccal side is characteristic of mandibular first primary molar. The buccal curvature of maxillary first primary molar is not as prominent as mandibular first primary molar.

11. Clinical emergence of a tooth occurs when:

(*a*) one-fourth of the root formation is complete

(*b*) one-half of the root formation is complete
(*c*) three-fourths of the root formation is complete
(*d*) root formation is complete

Answer (*c*).

According to Gron, tooth emergence appeared to be more closely associated with the stage of root formation than with the chronologic or skeletal age of the child. By the time of clinical emergence approximately three-fourths of root formation would have occurred. Teeth reach occlusion before the root development is complete.

12. According to Moyer, the most favorable sequence of eruption of maxillary permanent teeth is:

(*a*) 6, 1, 2, 4, 3, 5, 7 (*b*) 6, 1, 2, 3, 4, 5, 7
(*c*) 6, 1, 2, 4, 5, 3, 7 (*d*) 6, 1, 2, 5, 4, 3, 7

Answer (*c*).

In the maxillary arch, the first premolar ideally should erupt before the second premolar and they should be followed by the canine. The untimely loss of the primary molars in the maxillary arch, allowing the first permanent molar to drift and tip mesially, will result in the permanent canine being blocked out of the arch, usually to the labial side. The position of the developing second molar in the maxillary arch and it's relationship to the first permanent molar should be given special attention. Its eruption before the premolars and canine can cause a loss of arch length just as in the mandibular arch.

13. The most favourable eruption sequence for mandibular permanent teeth is:

(*a*) 6, 1, 2, 3, 4, 5, 7 (*b*) 6, 1, 2, 4, 5, 3, 7
(*c*) 6, 1, 3, 2, 4, 5, 7 (*d*) 6, 1, 2, 3, 7, 4, 5

Answer (*a*).

The most favourable sequence in mandibular arch is first permanent molar, central incisors, lateral incisors, canines, first and second premolars. It is desirable that the mandibular canine erupts before the first and second premolars. This sequence will aid in maintaining adequate arch length and in preventing lingual tipping of the incisors. Lingual tipping of the incisors not only will cause a loss of arch length but also will allow the development of an increased overbite.

14. Eruption sequestrum is made of:

(*a*) a tiny spicule of non viable bone

(*b*) dentin and cementum

(*c*) either osteogenic or odontogenic tissue

(*d*) any of the above

Answer (*d*).

Eruption sequestrum is defined as a tiny spicule of non-viable bone overlying the crown of an erupting permanent molar just before or immediately after the emergence of the tips of the cusps through the oral mucosa. It can be also composed of dentin, cementum, osteogenic or odontogenic tissue.

15. Among the primary teeth, the problem of ankylosis is most commonly seen with:

(*a*) mandibular molars

(*b*) mandibular incisors

(*c*) maxillary incisors

(*d*) maxillary molars

Answer (*a*).

Ankylosis is most commonly seen in mandibular molars among the primary teeth. Metallic sound on percussion is diagnostic of ankylosed and traumatically intruded teeth. Ankylosed teeth are also called submerged teeth.

16. All are features of a Mongoloid child except:

(*a*) bridge of the nose is depressed

(*b*) mental retardation

(*c*) delayed eruption of primary teeth

(*d*) eyes slope downward

Answer (*d*).

All the above mentioned features are common to Down Syndrome children except that the eyes of these children slope upwards.

17. All of the following conditions are associated with delayed eruption of teeth except:

(*a*) hyperthyroidism

(*b*) hypopituitarism

(*c*) cleidocranial dysplasia

(*d*) Gardner's syndrome

Answer (*a*).

In hyperthyroidism premature eruption of teeth is noticed. In hypopituitarism delayed eruption of teeth is seen. In severe cases, primary teeth do not exfoliate. The underlying permanent teeth also do not erupt. In some cases of cleidocranial dysplasia primary teeth are retained till 15 years of age. Gardner's syndrome is also associated with delayed eruption of teeth.

18. Maxillary diastema frequently do not close until the eruption of permanent:

(*a*) maxillary lateral incisors

(*b*) mandibular cuspids

(*c*) maxillary cuspids

(*d*) maxillary premolars

Answer (*c*).

In the mixed dentition physiologic spacing between incisors is normal because of the eruption pattern of permanent teeth. When the canines erupt, all the spaces will close. No treatment should be initiated if there is a possibility that the diastema is physiologic or if the canines have not erupted. Abnormal diastema may also result from supernumerary or missing teeth, oral habits, macroglossia or frenulae. Hence, an accurate diagnosis is necessary before treatment is initiated.

19. The crowns of all permanent teeth with the exception of third molars are calcified by the age of:

(*a*) 6 years (*b*) 8 years

(*c*) 12 years (*d*) 16 years

Answer (*b*).

The enamel formation of all permanent teeth except third molars is completed by 8 years of age. Hence, drugs like tetracycline which can cause discoloration of teeth should not be given until then.

20. The chronological age of a child is:

(*a*) closely related to the physiological age

(*b*) closely related to the dental age

(*c*) closely related to the skeletal age

(*d*) independent of the dental and skeletal ages

Answer (*d*).

Chronological age is not related to dental, physiological or skeletal ages. It is the most obvious and easily determined developmental age which is simply figured from the child's date of birth. The skeletal and the dental ages are based on the skeletal and dental development respectively.

21. In a normal child, the teeth that are generally in the process of calcification at birth are:

(*a*) all primary teeth only

(*b*) all primary teeth and first permanent molars

(*c*) primary anteriors, canines and first primary molars only

(*d*) all primary teeth and all permanent teeth

Answer (*b*).

All the primary teeth and the first permanent molars are in the process of calcification at birth.

22. A radiograph of a 4-year-old child reveals no evidence of calcification of mandibular second premolars. This means that:

(*a*) these teeth may develop later

(*b*) the child will probably never develop second premolars

(*c*) it is too early in life to make any predictions concerning the development of any permanent tooth

(*d*) extraction of primary second molar should be performed to allow the permanent first molars to drift forward

Answer (*a*).

The hard tissue formation of mandibular second premolars begins between 2.25 to 2.5 years. Sometimes it can be delayed and may start after 4 years also. Hence extraction of second primary molar should not be performed.

23. A disturbance during the calcification stage of tooth development is the cause of:

(*a*) peg teeth

(*b*) microdontia

(*c*) oligodontia

(*d*) interglobular dentin

Answer (*d*).

Disturbance during the calcification stage can result in interglobular dentin formation. Refer to the explanation of Q. No. 2.

24. Tooth buds generally initiated after birth include:

(*a*) entire permanent dentition only

(*b*) all permanent teeth and some primary teeth

(*c*) 1st, 2nd premolars and second and third molars only

(*d*) all primary teeth

Answer (*c*).

All the primary teeth buds are initiated in the intrauterine period itself whereas the tooth buds generally initiated after birth include 1st, 2nd premolar, 2nd, and 3rd molars. Hard tissue formation begins at birth for the first permanent molars and in the intrauterine period itself for all primary teeth.

Chapter 3

Child Psychology

1. A child aged 4 would be classified developmentally according to Stone and Church as a:

(*a*) toddler

(*b*) preschooler

(*c*) middle year child

(*d*) adoloscent

Answer (*b*).

Stone and Church's classification:

Infant	–	Till 15 months
Toddler	–	5 months to 2 years of age
Preschooler	–	2 to 6 years of age
Middle year child	–	6 to 12 years of age
Adolescent	–	12 years till maturity

2. A two-year-old preschooler shows active happy hustle-bustle type of reception-room behaviour. His most likely response to oral examination will be:

(*a*) definitely negative

(*b*) negative

(*c*) positive to modelling

(*d*) positive to effective communication

Answer (*b*).

A two-year-old child is classified by Wright as: too young to cooperate. Hence the response to oral examination will invariably be negative.

3. When a patient is exposed step by step in a hierarchy from the least to the most stressful procedures repeatedly until there is no evidence of stress, the procedure is known as:

(*a*) modelling (*b*) restraining

(*c*) desensitization (*d*) reinforcement

Answer (*c*).

This procedure is known as desensitization. Systematic desensitization as a behaviour modification procedure uses two important elements:

(*a*) Gradational exposure of the child to his or her fear.

(*b*) Induced state of incompatibility with his or her own fear.

4. Approving a child's behaviour in front of its parents verbally is known as:

(*a*) social (*b*) material

(*c*) activity (*d*) none of the above

Answer (a).

Praise, positive facial expressions, nearness, and physical contact come under social reinforcers and they represent the majority of all reinforcing events.

5. Which of the following is not a part of Erikson's model for personality development?

(*a*) Trust versus Mistrust

(*b*) Initiative versus Guilt

(*c*) Autonomy versus Doubt

(*d*) None of the above

Answer (*d*).

All the above mentioned concepts are a part of Erikson's psychosocial theory.

6. When a child is complemented or rewarded in some manner for his or her cooperative behaviour, it is known as:

(*a*) punishment

(*b*) restrainment

(*c*) positive reinforcement

(*d*) negative reinforcement

Answer (*c*).

If a pleasant consequence follows a response, the response has been positively reinforced and the behaviour, that led to this pleasant consequence becomes more likely in the future dental visits.

7. Id, ego and superego are part of:

(*a*) Freud's psychoanalytical theory

(*b*) Erikson's model of personality development

(*c*) Piaget's theory

(*d*) Skinner's theory

Answer (*a*).

Id, ego and superego are components of Sigmund Freud's psychoanalytical theory.

S. No.	*Components*	*Description*	*Principle*
1.	Id	Id is defined as the inherited reservoir of unorganized drives, it is mostly unconscious, is governed by the pleasure-pain principle, aims at immediate satisfaction of libidinal urges, is immoral, illogical and lacks unity of purpose.	Pleasure-pain principle
2.	Ego	Ego is defined as the integrating or mediating part of personality, which develops out of interaction of id and environment. It has perception of both the internal and the external world.	Reality principle
3.	Super ego	Superego is defined as the latest development of the mind embodying the code of society and including concepts of right and wrong, the value system and the ideals.	

8. Preventive desensitization means:

(*a*) behaviour shaping

(*b*) tell, show, do procedures

(*c*) graded introduction of child to dentistry

(*d*) all of the above

Answer (*d*).

All these techniques are effective methods of managing child behaviour during initial and subsequent dental visits.

9. A child's behaviour problem in the dental office can be handled by familiarization if the basis of the problem is:

(*a*) the parents (*b*) pain

(*c*) emotional (*d*) fear

Answer (*d*).

The answer is self-explanatory.

10. The basic fear of most children under 2 years of age is concerned with:

(*a*) separation from the parent

(*b*) injection of local anesthetics

(*c*) the reason for dental treatment

(*d*) the instruments to perform dental treatment

Answer (*a*).

The basic fear of most children under the age of 2 years is separation anxiety.

Chapter 4

Behaviour Management

1. Pedodontic treatment triangle was given by:

(*a*) G.Z. Wright

(*b*) Henry Kempe

(*c*) Evangeline Jordan

(*d*) Addleston

Answer (*a*).

G.Z. Wright introduced the pedodontic treatment triangle. Henry Kempe introduced the term battered-child syndrome. Evangeline Jordan introduced hand-over-mouth exercise. Addleston introduced TSD (tell show and do) technique.

2. Which of the following is correct about the pedodontic treatment triangle?

(*a*) Child is at the apex of the triangle.

(*b*) The arrows placed on the lines of the triangle indicate that the communication is reciprocal.

(*c*) This triangle illustrates the 1:2 relationship in pediatric dentistry.

(*d*) All of the above.

Answer (*d*).

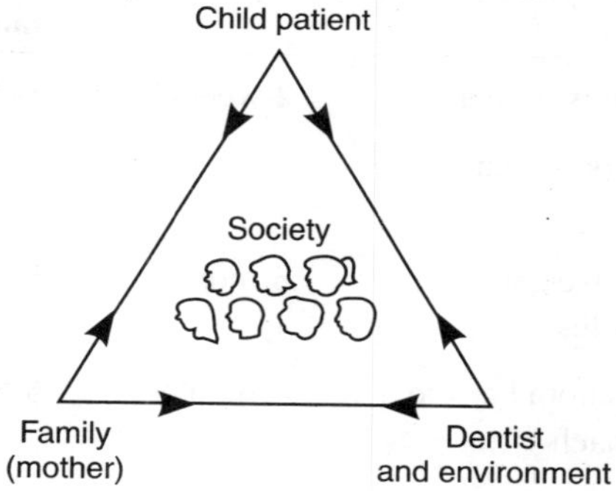

Fig. 4.1 Pedodontic treatment triangle.

As the child is the primary focus in pediatric dentistry, he or she is placed at the apex of the triangle. The communication is between the child and dentist, dentist and parent, and parent and child, which is indicated by arrows on the triangle. As the dentist communicates with both the child and the parents it is a 1:2 relationship. On the other hand, in adult dentistry the dentist communicates only with the patient (1:1 relationship).

3. The average age range by which a child stands alone is:

(*a*) 3–4 months

(*b*) 9–18 months

(*c*) 20–24 months

(*d*) 1–2 months

Answer (*b*).

Average age range of selected physical developmental milestones

S. No.	*Developmental task*	*Average age*	*Normal range*
1.	Focuses on light	2 weeks	1–4 weeks
2.	Lies on stomach, lifts chin	3 weeks	1–10 weeks
3.	Birth weight doubles	6 months	5–7 months
4.	Rolls from back to stomach	7 months	5½–11 months
5.	Sits alone	7 months	6–11 months
6.	Stands with support	10 months	7½–14 months
7.	Stands alone	13½ months	9–18 months
8.	Walks alone	14 months	10–20 months
9.	Attains bowel control	18 months	1–2½ years
10.	First menstruation (in girls)	12 years 9 months	10–17 years

4. The intelligence quotient (IQ) concept was measured by Alfred Binet by primarily examining which of the following tasks?

(*a*) Memory

(*b*) Spatial relationship

(*c*) Reasoning

(*d*) All of the above

Answer (*d*).

The answer is self-explanatory.

5. The IQ formula used by Binet was:

(*a*) $$\text{IQ} = \frac{\text{Mental age}}{\text{Chronologic age}} \times 100$$

(*b*) $$\text{IQ} = \frac{\text{Chronologic age}}{\text{Mental age}} \times 100$$

(*c*) $$\text{IQ} = \frac{\text{Chronologic age}}{\text{Dental age}} \times 100$$

(*d*) $$\text{IQ} = \frac{\text{Skeletal age}}{\text{Chronologic age}} \times 100$$

Answer (*a*).

The answer is self-explanatory.

6. According to American Association of Mental Deficiency classification, which of the following descriptions describes "mild" mental retardation?

(*a*) Can be educated in special classes to gain elementary school level academic skills

(*b*) Can be trained to perform self-help skills and to achieve sheltered workshop employment

(*c*) Abilities typically limited to simple language usage and the mastery of basic self-help skills

(*d*) Consistent custodial care required

Answer (*a*).

American Association of Mental Deficiency Classification

S. No.	*IQ range*	*Description*	*Practical description*
1.	52–68	Mild	Can be educated in special classes to gain elementary school-level academic skills
2.	36–51	Moderate	Can be trained to perform self-help skills and to achieve sheltered workshop employment
3.	20–35	Severe	Abilities typically limited to simple language usage and the masters of basic self-help skills
4.	19 and below	Profound	Consistent custodial care required

7. A child visits the dental clinic, has a good rapport with the dentist, is interested in the dental procedures, is laughing and enjoying the treatment. According to Frankl what is the rating given for this behaviour?

(*a*) Rating 1 (*b*) Rating 2

(*c*) Rating 3 (*d*) Rating 4

Answer (*d*).

Frankl behaviour rating scale:

Rating 1—Definitely negative—Refusal of treatment, crying forcefully, fearful or any other avert evidence of extreme negativism.

Rating 2—Negative—Reluctant to accept treatment, uncooperative, some evidence of negative attitude but not pronounced (sullen, withdrawn).

Rating 3—Positive—Acceptance of treatment, at times cautious, willing to comply with the dentist, at times with reservation, but the patient follows the dentist's directions.

Rating 4—Definitely positive—Good rapport with the dentist, interested in dental procedures, laughing and enjoying.

8. A child of 2 years of age reports to the dental office with its parents and resists examination by the dentist. According to Wright's classification of child's behaviour which category the child will fall in?

(*a*) Cooperative

(*b*) Lacking cooperative ability

(*c*) Potentially cooperative

(*d*) Timid behaviour

Answer (*b*).

Wright's classification of child behaviour:

A. **Cooperative**—Most children in the dental office cooperate.

B. **Lacking cooperative ability**

1. Children with whom communication cannot be established and comprehension cannot be expected (children less than 3 years of age).
2. Those children who lack cooperative ability because of debilitating or disabling condition.

C. **Potentially cooperative**—In this category the child's behavior can be modified and the child can become cooperative. This is further classified into—uncontrolled, defiant, timid, tense cooperative, whining and stoic behaviour.

9. Which of the following statements is true?

(*a*) Pre-appointment behaviour modification refers to anything that is said or done to positively influence the child's behaviour before the child enters the operatory.

(*b*) In recent years pre-appointment behaviour modification is done with audio-visual aids for modelling and pre-appointment mailings.

(*c*) This strategy prepares the pediatric patient in advance and makes the first dental visit pleasant.

(*d*) All the above statements are true.

Answer (*d*).

The answer is self-explanatory.

10. Behaviour shaping is a form of behaviour modification. It is based on the established principles of social learning.

(*a*) Both the statements are true.

(*b*) Both the statements are false.

(*c*) First statement is true and the second is false.

(*d*) First statement is false and the second is true.

Answer (*a*).

Behaviour shaping is that procedure which very slowly develops behaviour by reinforcing successive approximations of the desired behaviour.

11. TSD was introduced by:

(*a*) Le Vitas (*b*) Wright

(*c*) Addleston (*d*) Gesell

Answer (*c*).

Addleston in 1959 first described the TSD (tell, show and do) technique. This technique addresses the anxiety of the child and provides acceptable means to cope with it by making the "unknown" known to the child (by telling, showing and doing).

12. HOME was introduced by:

(*a*) Le Vitas (*b*) Evangeline Jordan

(*c*) Addelston (*d*) Gesell

Answer (*b*).

This technique was first described by Dr. Evangeline Jordan in 1920 and she named it hand-over-mouth technique. Le Vitas renamed this technique as HOME (Hand-over-mouth exercise).

13. The primary objective of HOME and voice control is:

(*a*) to gain the attention of a highly oppositional child so that communication can be established

(*b*) to do filling in the same appointment

(*c*) to make the child understand that improper behaviour will lead to punishment

(*d*) to prepare the child for eventual extraction

Answer (*a*).

HOME and voice control are used to manage children showing disruptive behaviour. When a child is crying uncontrollably these methods are used to muffle the noise so that the dentist can convey whatever has to be conveyed.

14. Aversive conditioning (HOME) is not used routinely but as a method of last resort, in children who have appropriate communicative abilities in the age group of:

(*a*) 2–3 years (*b*) 3–6 years

(*c*) 9–12 years (*d*) 12–15 years

Asnwer (*b*).

A child less than 3 years of age may cry even more forcefully when voice control is used. Hence, these techniques are used only in children of the 3–6 years age group.

15. A bribe is promised to induce the desired behaviour. A reward is recognition of good behaviour after the completion of the operation, without previously implied promise (by FINN):

(*a*) both the statements are true

(*b*) both the statements are false

(*c*) first statement is true and the second is false

(*d*) first statement is false and the second is true

Answer (*a*).

The question explains the difference between a bribe and a reward.

Chapter 5

Pharmacological Behaviour Management of Children

1. Which of the following statements will you take into account when a child patient is posted for dental treatment under general anesthesia?

(*a*) Narrow airway in children.

(*b*) Children have reduced tolerance to airway obstruction.

(*c*) Cardiovascular parameters are different for a child.

(*d*) All of the above.

Answer (*d*).

In a pediatric patient, narrow nasal passages and glottis combined with hypertrophic tonsils and adenoids, enlarged tongue and greater secretion produce a greater risk of airway obstruction. Because of their reduced tolerance to respiratory obstruction sudden apnea is a great concern. The heart rate is faster and the blood pressure is lower than the adult patient.

2. Which of the following is not true of conscious sedation?

(*a*) A pharmacologically induced controlled state.

(*b*) Minimally depressed level of consciousness.

(*c*) Ability to maintain airway independently and continuously.

(*d*) Inability to respond to physical stimuli and verbal command.

Answer (*d*).

Conscious sedation is defined as a controlled, pharmacologically induced, minimally depressed level of consciousness, in which the patient retains the ability to maintain airway independently and continuously and responds to physical stimuli and verbal command.

3. All of the following are true regarding deep sedation except:

(*a*) controlled state induced pharmacologically

(*b*) patient not easily aroused

(*c*) partial loss of protective reflexes

(*d*) minimally depressed consciousness

Answer (*d*).

Deep sedation is defined as controlled, pharmacologically induced, deeply depressed level of consciousness, a state in which there is partial loss of protective reflexes from which the patient is not easily aroused.

4. Which of the following is true regarding general anesthesia?

(*a*) Pharmacologically induced state.

(*b*) State of unconsciousness.

(*c*) Partial or complete loss of reflexes.

(*d*) All of the above.

Answer (*d*).

General anesthesia is a pharmacologically induced state of unconsciousness where there is partial or complete loss of reflexes.

5. Which of the following is an indication for conscious sedation?

(*a*) Patient who cannot understand or cooperate.

(*b*) Patient who cannot cooperate because of lack of psychological maturity.

(*c*) Patient who cannot cooperate because of cognitive, physical or medical disability.

(*d*) All of the above.

Answer (*d*).

The answer is self-explanatory.

6. Which of the following is a requisite for sedation procedures?

(*a*) Informed consent.

(*b*) Careful patient evaluation and availability of emergency services.

(*c*) Knowledge of agents used.

(*d*) All of the above.

Answer (*d*).

All of the above mentioned factors are requisites for sedation procedures.

7. The most commonly used routes for sedation are:

(*a*) inhalational, oral and intravenous

(*b*) inhalational, oral and submucosal

(*c*) intramuscular, intravenous and oral

(*d*) intravenous, oral and rectal

Answer (*a*).

Sedative drugs may be administered through inhalational, oral, rectal, submucosal, intramuscular or intravenous routes. But the most commonly used routes are inhalational, oral and intravenous.

8. Which of the following is not an objective of conscious sedation?

(*a*) Patient's mood should be altered.

(*b*) Child should remain unconscious.

(*c*) All vital signs should be stable.

(*d*) Pain threshold should be elevated.

Answer (*b*).

In conscious sedation the patient should be conscious. Refer to the explanation of Q. No. 2.

9. Which of the following is an objective of conscious sedation?

(*a*) Amnesia should occur.

(*b*) To provide most efficient high-quality dental care.

(*c*) To provide positive psychologic attitude.

(*d*) All of the above.

Answer (*d*).

The primary objective of these techniques is to produce a quiescent patient to ensure the best quality of care and to help train a child to willingly accept, future dental care.

10. The most commonly used agent for inhalational conscious sedation is:

(*a*) Nitrous oxide-oxygen

(*b*) Halothane

(*c*) Ether

(*d*) Fluorothane

Answer (*a*).

Nitrous oxide-oxygen is the most commonly used inhalational sedating agent. All the other agents mentioned above are general anesthesia agents.

11. One of the primary advantages of inhalational route in conscious sedation is:

(*a*) sedation can be reversed at any moment

(*b*) drug absorption is less

(*c*) post-operative complications are less

(*d*) patient tolerance is good

Answer (*a*).

Sedation can be reversed at any moment by withdrawing the mask and thereby introducing nitrous oxide-oxygen into the system.

12. Nitrous oxide is:

(*a*) colourless

(*b*) slightly sweet smelling

(*c*) heavier than air

(*d*) all of the above

Answer (*d*).

Nitrous oxide is slightly heavier than air with a specific gravity of 1.53. It has a blood-gas partition coefficient of 0.47. Because of its low solubility in blood it has a very rapid onset and recovery time.

13. Which of the following statements are false regarding nitrous oxide administration for conscious sedation?

(*a*) It is physically dissolved in the serum fraction of the blood.

(*b*) Nitrous oxide has a minimum alveolar concentration of 105.

(*c*) It has chemical combination with the blood components.

(*d*) When the concentration gradient is reversed, the gas is rapidly excreted by the lungs.

Answer (*c*).

Nitrous oxide is physically dissolved in blood but has no chemical combination with any of the blood components. Also it does not undergo any biotransformation.

14. Nitrous oxide-oxygen anesthesia can cause:

(*a*) hypoxic hypoxia

(*b*) diffusion hypoxia

(*c*) nitrous hypoxia

(*d*) hypoxia with cyanosis

Answer (*b*).

A phenomenon termed diffusion hypoxia may occur as the sedation is reversed at the termination of the procedure. Nitrous oxide escapes into the alveoli rapidly so that the oxygen present in the alveoli becomes diluted. The oxygen-carbon dioxide exchange is disrupted and a period of hypoxia is created. This is termed as diffusion hypoxia, which can be minimized by oxygenation for about 5 minutes after the sedation procedure.

15. When does diffusion hypoxia occur during the conscious-sedation procedure?

(*a*) At the beginning of the procedure.

(*b*) At the end of the procedure.

(*c*) In between the procedure.

(*d*) Five minutes after starting the procedure.

Answer (*b*).

Diffusion hypoxia may occur as the sedation is reversed at the termination of the procedure. However this phenomenon is reported not to occur in healthy pediatric patients.

16. The side effects of nitrous oxide exposure for prolonged periods include:

(*a*) high rates of spontaneous abortion

(*b*) neurotoxicity

(*c*) hepatotoxicity

(*d*) all of the above

Answer (*d*).

Chronic exposure to nitrous oxide can produce recreational abuse, neurotoxicity, impotence, renal and liver toxicity, higher rate of spontaneous abortions and decrease in fertility.

17. Which of the following is true of nitrous oxide-oxygen sedation?

(*a*) It causes an altered state of awareness.

(*b*) It is a CNS depressant.

(*c*) It produces limited analgesia.

(*d*) All of the above.

Answer (*d*).

All of the above mentioned factors are true regarding nitrous oxide-oxygen sedation.

18. First step after placing the mask in nitrous oxide sedation procedure is:

(*a*) administering 30% nitrous oxide and 70% oxygen

(*b*) administering 50% nitrous oxide and 50% oxygen

(*c*) administering 100% oxygen

(*d*) administering 70% nitrous oxide and 30% oxygen

Answer (*c*).

First, the bag is filled with 100% oxygen and delivered to the patient for 2–3 minutes at an appropriate slow rate typically between 4–6 liters per minute. Then nitrous oxide can be introduced in slowly increasing concentrations (at increments of 10–20%) to achieve the desired level.

19. Maintenance dose of nitrous oxide-oxygen for conscious sedation is:

(*a*) Nitrous oxide 70% and oxygen 30%

(*b*) Nitrous oxide 30% and oxygen 70%

(*c*) Nitrous oxide 50% and oxygen 50%

(*d*) Nitrous oxide 80% and oxygen 20%

Answer (*b*).

The patient can be maintained at 30% nitrous oxide and 70% oxygen or lower and monitored and the contemplated procedure can be carried out.

20. To prevent diffusion hypoxia after nitrous oxide-oxygen sedation:

(*a*) 100% oxygen is administered for 5 minutes

(*b*) 100% oxygen is administered for 30 minutes

(*c*) nitrous oxide-oxygen concentration is reduced gradually

(*d*) 70% oxygen is administered for 5 minutes

Answer (*a*).

To minimize the effect of diffusion hypoxia, the patient should be oxygenated with 100% oxygen for 5 minutes after the sedation procedure.

21. Which of the following is an indication that the patient is adequately sedated?

(*a*) Floating sensation and giddy feeling.

(*b*) Tingling sensation of digits.

(*c*) Distant gaze or sagging eyelids.

(*d*) Any of the above.

Answer (*d*).

All the above mentioned features indicate that the patient is adequately sedated.

22. The dentist who used nitrous oxide for the first time is:

(*a*) Colton (*b*) Horace Wells

(*c*) Long (*d*) Priestley

Answer (*b*).

The answer is self-explanatory.

23. Whose demonstration of properties of nitrous oxide instigated Horace Wells to use nitrous oxide for tooth extraction?

(*a*) Colton (*b*) Horace Wells

(*c*) Long (*d*) Priestley

Answer (*a*).

Colton's (a physicist) demonstration of properties of nitrous oxide instigated Horace Wells to use nitrous oxide for tooth extraction.

24. All of the following anti-histamine drugs are used for conscious sedation except:

(*a*) hydroxyzine (*b*) promethazine

(*c*) chlorpromazine (*d*) meperidine

Answer (*d*).

Meperdine being a narcotic drug cannot be used for conscious sedation.

25. One of the following agents is used for sedation only by inhalational route:

(*a*) halothane

(*b*) nitrous oxide-oxygen

(*c*) promethazine

(*d*) Isofluorane

Answer (*b*).

Nitrous oxide-oxygen is used for sedation only through inhalational route. Halothane and Isoflurane are general anesthetic agents. Promethazine is a phenothiazine with sedative and anti-histaminic properties.

26. One of the following benzodiazepines is frequently used nowadays for conscious sedation:

(*a*) diazepam (*b*) midazolam

(*c*) hydroxyzine (*d*) fentanyl

Answer (*b*).

Midazolam is used as an intravenous sedative agent. It is a benzodiazepine group of drug. After intravenous administration, sedation occurs in 3–5 minutes.

27. Which of the following conditions in a 6-year-old patient is a contraindication to the use of nitrous oxide-oxygen analgesia?

(*a*) The child has cold.

(*b*) The child is mentally retarded.

(*c*) The child has a history of diabetes.

(*d*) The child is allergic to local anesthesia.

Answer (*a*).

The answer is self-explanatory.

28. Which of the following intravenous agents is commonly used as an induction agent?

(*a*) Diazepam

(*b*) Ketamine

(*c*) Thiopental

(*d*) Phenobarbitone

Answer (*c*).

Thiopental and Methohexital are ultra-short acting barbiturates commonly used as induction agents.

29. Commonly used drug combination for oral sedation is:

(*a*) Chloralhydrate + Hydroxyzine

(*b*) Chloralhydrate + Hydroxyzine + Meperidine

(*c*) Meperidine + Hydroxyzine

(*d*) Any of the above

Answer (*d*).

All of the above mentioned drug combinations are used for oral sedation.

30. Which of the following routes are titrable?

(*a*) I.V. and inhalational

(*b*) I.V. and I.M.

(*c*) I.V. and oral

(*d*) Oral and subcutaneous

Answer (*a*).

I.V. and inhalational routes are titrable.

31. Which of the following is a contraindication for conscious sedation?

(*a*) If medical history reveals him or her to be a high-risk patient.

(*b*) Pregnancy.

(*c*) ASA III and IV group patient.

(*d*) All of the above.

Answer (*d*).

The answer is self-explanatory. Refer to the table below.

American Society of Anesthesiologists classification

S. No.	*Class*	*Description*
1.	Class I	There is no organic, physiologic, biochemical or psychiatric disturbance. The pathologic process for which operation is to be performed is localized and is not a systemic disturbance.
2.	Class II	Mild to moderate systemic disturbance caused either by the condition to be treated surgically or by other pathophysiologic processes.
3.	Class III	Severe systemic disturbance or disease.
4.	Class IV	Indicative of the patient with severe systemic disorders that are already life threatening.
5.	Class V	The moribund patient who has little chance of survival without the planned procedure.

32. Which drug should be available if Meperidine is used for premedication?

(*a*) Atropine (*b*) Naloxone

(*c*) Promethazine (*d*) Lactamine

Answer (*b*).

Meperidine is a narcotic agent. When it is used for premedication, narcotic antagonist Naloxone should be available.

33. The nitrous oxide administered for conscious sedation in a patient:

(*a*) gets excreted by the kidneys

(*b*) is detoxified in the liver

(*c*) is exhaled by lungs

(*d*) is metabolized to nitrous oxide and oxygen

Answer (*c*).

Nitrous oxide does not combine chemically with blood components. Hence it is just exhaled by the lungs.

34. A child who has been given a sedative dose of barbiturate (short acting) is active and excited. This indicates:

(*a*) normal response to the drug

(*b*) excessive dose of drug

(*c*) insufficient dose of drug

(*d*) unexpected reaction

Answer (*c*).

If the dose is insufficient, barbiturates can cause excitement in children instead of sedation.

Chapter 6

Nutrition and Dental Health

1. Deficiency of which of the following causes neural tube defects like anencephaly and spina bifida?

(*a*) Iron (*b*) Folic acid

(*c*) Zinc (*d*) Calcium

Answer (*b*).

Folic acid deficiency causes neural tube defects like anencephaly and spina bifida.

2. The amount of folic acid required for prevention of neural tube defects is approximately:

(*a*) 100–200 μg/day

(*b*) 200–250 μg/day

(*c*) 200–400 μg/day

(*d*) more than 600 μg/day

Answer (*c*).

The amount of folic acid required to prevent neural tube defects is 200–400 μg/day.

3. Zinc deficiency can cause:

(*a*) dwarfism

(*b*) hypogonadism

(*c*) delayed sexual maturation

(*d*) any of the above

Answer (*d*).

Zinc plays an important role in growth and development. This trace element is also required for proper wound healing. Severe deficiencies result in dwarfism, hypogonadism, and delayed sexual maturation.

4. The daily dietary recommendation of calcium in children is:

(*a*) 600–800 mg (*b*) 800–1200 mg

(*c*) 1200–1600 mg (*d*) 1600–2000 mg

Answer (*b*).

The daily dietary recommendation of calcium in children is 800–1200 mg.

5. Anorexia nervosa is characterized by self-imposed weight loss, amenorrhea and distorted attitude towards eating and body weight. Binge eating and invariably self-induced vomiting characterize bulimia nervosa.

(*a*) Both the statements are false.

(*b*) Both the statements are true.

(*c*) First statement is true and the second is false.

(*d*) First statement is false and the second is true.

Answer (*b*).

During adolescence or before, some individuals (primarily girls) become preoccupied with their appearance and body weight and as a result restrict their food intake. Anorexia nervosa results when this behaviour is carried to the point of starvation. Bulimia nervosa is characterized by self-induced vomiting and it is more common than anorexia nervosa.

6. Enamel erosion is common among bulimia-nervosa patients. Fluoxetine hydrochloride appears to help control the obsessive-compulsive behaviour involved in both anorexia nervosa and bulimia nervosa.

(*a*) Both the statements are false.

(*b*) Both the statements are true.

(*c*) First statement is true and the second is false.

(*d*) First statement is false and the second is true.

Answer (*b*).

Enamel erosion is common in patients with bulimia nervosa because of the exposure of the tooth surfaces to the highly acidic regurgitated gastric contents. Anti-depressants may be helpful in some cases.

7. The immature kidneys of a baby cannot concentrate waste efficiently. As a result the infant must excrete relatively more water than an adult to eliminate a comparable amount of waste.

(*a*) Both the statements are false.

(*b*) Both the statements are true.

(*c*) First statement is true and the second is false.

(*d*) First statement is false and the second is true.

Answer (*b*).

The answer is self-explanatory. However, when dealing with infants, one must be careful of dehydration which has potentially serious consequences.

8. The most rapid growth occurs in humans during:

(*a*) prenatal period
(*b*) 6–12 months of age
(*c*) between 3–5 years of life
(*d*) beginning of teenage years

Answer (*a*).

Prenatal period shows the most rapid growth in humans. The next rapid growth occurs during the first six months of life.

9. All the following statements are true except:

(*a*) atherosclerosis begins early in life
(*b*) atherosclerosis of coronary arteries can produce myocardial infarction and coronary heart disease
(*c*) atherosclerosis is positively associated with elevated HDL (high density lipoprotein) levels
(*d*) hypercholesterolemia, hypertension and cigarette smoking are the three major risk factors for coronary heart disease

Answer (*c*).

Atherosclerosis is negatively associated with elevated HDL concentrations and positively associated with elevated total serum cholesterol and elevated LDL (low density lipoprotein) levels. A prudent health goal will be to reduce the elevated levels of total and LDL cholesterol and increase the HDL levels.

10. Diagnostic criteria for anorexia nervosa includes all the following except:

(*a*) self-induced weight loss leading to maintenance of body weight less than 85% of that expected
(*b*) intense fear of weight gain

(*c*) Recurrent episodes of binge eating

(*d*) Endocrine changes manifesting as amenorrhoea in females

Answer (*c*).

Recurrent episodes of binge eating followed by self-induced vomiting or use of laxatives is diagnostic of bulimia nervosa.

Chapter 7

Dental Caries and Fluorides

1. The most widely accepted theory of the cause of dental caries is:

(*a*) Proteolysis-chelation theory

(*b*) Proteolysis theory

(*c*) Acidogenic theory or chemicoparasitic theory

(*d*) Hypoplastic theory

Answer (*c*).

The most popular and probably the most widely accepted theory is Miller's acidogenic theory. Refer to the table below for description of theories.

S. No.	*Name of the theory*	*Author*	*Description*
1.	Chemicoparasitic or acidogenic	Miller	Dental caries is caused by acids resulting from the action of microorganisms on carbohydrates. It is characterized by decalcification of inorganic portion and is accompanied or

			followed by disintegration of the organic substance of the tooth.
2.	Proteolysis theory	Gottlieb and Frisbie	Dental caries is caused by microorganisms which invade enamel lamellae and involve the dentin.
3.	Proteolysis chelation theory	Schatz	Oral bacteria attack organic components of enamel and the break-down products have chelating ability, which dissolve the tooth minerals.

2. Oral bacteria attacks organic components of enamel and the breakdown products have the ability to dissolve the tooth minerals. This is:

(*a*) proteolysis-chelation theory

(*b*) proteolysis theory

(*c*) acidogenic theory or chemicoparasitic theory

(*d*) hypoplastic theory

Answer (*a*).

Refer to the explanation of Q. No. 1.

3. Proteolysis theory was proposed by:

(*a*) Miller

(*b*) Gottlieb and Frisbie

(*c*) Fitzerald

(*d*) Keyes

Answer (*b*).

Refer to the explanation of Q. No. 1.

4. Acids resulting from the action of microorganisms on carbohydrates cause dental caries, which is characterized by decalcification of inorganic portion and followed by disintegration of organic substances. This theory is:

(*a*) proteolysis-chelation theory

(*b*) proteolysis theory

(*c*) acidogenic theory or chemicoparasitic theory

(*d*) hypoplastic theory

Answer (*c*).

Refer to the explanation of Q. No. 1.

5. Animals maintained in a germ-free environment did not develop caries even when fed on a high carbohydrate diet. This was proven by:

(*a*) Miller

(*b*) Gottlieb

(*c*) Orland and Fitzerald

(*d*) Loesche

Answer (*c*).

Studies by Orland and by Fitzerald, Jordan and Achard demonstrated that dental caries will not occur in the absence of microorganisms. Animals maintained in a germ-free environment did not develop caries even when fed a high-carbohydrate diet. However, dental caries did develop in these animals when they were inoculated with microorganisms from caries-active animals and then fed cariogenic diets.

6. Streptococcus mutans is present in the oral cavity of infants at birth. Streptococcus mutans is transmitted orally from mother to infant.

(*a*) Both the statements are false.

(*b*) Both the statements are true.

(*c*) First statement is true and the second is false.

(*d*) First statement is false and the second is true.

Answer (*d*).

Streptococcus mutans is not present in the oral cavity of infants at birth and can be detected only after the primary teeth begin to erupt. Transmission of Streptococcus mutans from mother to infant is confirmed by many investigators.

7. The acids that initially decalcify the enamel have a pH of:

(*a*) 1–2 (*b*) 5.5–5.2

(*c*) 7–6.8 (*d*) 2–3

Answer (*b*).

The answer is self-explanatory.

8. Outer surface of enamel is far more resistant to demineralization by acids than deeper portion of enamel. Hence, the greatest amount of demineralization occurs 10–15 microns beneath the enamel surface.

(*a*) Both the statements are false.

(*b*) Both the statements are true.

(*c*) First statement is true and the second is false.

(*d*) First statement is false and the second is true.

Answer (*b*).

This demineralization that occurs 10–15 microns below the outer surface is called subsurface demineralization. The continuation of this process results in the subsurface enamel lesion that will first be observed as white spot lesion.

9. The time required for remineralization to replace the hydroxyapatite lost during demineralization is determined by:

(*a*) the age of the plaque

(*b*) nature of carbohydrate consumed

(*c*) presence or absence of fluoride

(*d*) all of the above.

Answer (d).

In the presence of dental plaque that has developed for 12 hours or less, the enamel demineralization resulting from a single exposure to sucrose will be remineralized by saliva within about 10 minutes. A period of at least 4 hours is required by saliva to repair the damage to enamel resulting from a similar exposure to sucrose in the presence of dental plaque that is 48 or more hours old. Presence of fluoride greatly enhances the rate of remineralization and also helps in formation of fluor-hydroxyapatite.

10. In the presence of dental plaque that has developed for 12 hours or less, the enamel demineralization resulting from a single exposure to sucrose will be remineralized by saliva within about.

(*a*) 10 minutes (*b*) 60 minutes

(*c*) 2 hours (*d*) 4 hours

Answer (a).

Refer to the explanation of Q. No. 9.

11. The organic acids that are usually involved in demineralization are:

(*a*) acetic acid (*b*) pyruvic acid

(*c*) lactic acid (*d*) (*a*) and (*b*)

(*e*) (*a*), (*b*) and (*c*)

Answer (*e*).

Demineralization is produced by weak organic acids such as lactic acid, acetic acid and pyruvic acid.

12. The second primary molar has deeper and less completely coalesced pits and fissures. This results in a higher susceptibility of second primary molar to dental caries, even though the first primary molar erupts earlier.

(*a*) Both the statements are false.

(*b*) Both the statements are true.

(*c*) First statement is true and the second is false.

(*d*) First statement is false and the second is true.

Answer (*b*).

The answer is self-explanatory.

13. Additional period required for enamel calcification after eruption is usually:

(*a*) 5 years (*b*) 1 year

(*c*) 2 years (*d*) 8 years

Answer (*c*).

Enamel calcification is incomplete at the time of eruption of the teeth and an additional period of about 2 years is required for the calcification process to be completed by exposure to saliva.

14. Which of the following secondary factors contribute to the etiology of dental caries?

(*a*) Anatomic characteristics of teeth.

(*b*) Arrangement of teeth in the arch.

(*c*) Presence of dental appliances.

(*d*) Hereditary factors.

(*e*) All of the above.

Answer (*e*).

Permanent molars often have incompletely coalesced pits and fissures that allow dental plaque material to be retained at the base of the defect in contact with exposed dentin. Crowded and irregular teeth are not readily cleansed during the masticatory process. Dental appliances increases the risk of decay by retaining more microorganisms. Tooth morphology and enamel defects tend to follow a familial pattern. Hence, heredity may play an indirect role by genetically producing caries susceptible surfaces.

15. Rampant caries is been defined as suddenly appearing, widespread, rapidly burrowing type of caries, resulting in early involvement of the pulp, affecting those teeth that are usually regarded as immune to tooth decay. This definition is given by:

(*a*) Massler (*b*) Fitzerald

(*c*) Keyes (*d*) Tinanoff

Answer (*a*).

The answer is self-explanatory.

16. Rampant caries can be caused by:

(*a*) high sucrose intake

(*b*) emotional disturbances

(*c*) patient under stress who takes tranquilizers and sedatives

(*d*) any of the above

Answer (*d*).

Repressed emotions and fears, dissatisfaction with achievement, rebellion against a home situation, a feeling of inferiority, a traumatic school experience and continuous general tension have been observed in children and adults who have rampant dental caries. An emotional disturbance may initiate an unusual craving for sweets which in turn influence the incidence of dental caries. Patients who take tranquilizers have decreased salivary flow resulting in lowered caries resistance.

17. The physical state of carbohydrates and the frequency of ingestion contribute to the initiation and extension of dental caries. Fermentable carbohydrates taken in an adherent form are more cariogenic than those consumed in soluble form.

(*a*) Both the statements are false.

(*b*) Both the statements are true.

(*c*) First statement is true and the second is false.

(*d*) First statement is false and the second is true.

Answer (*b*).

The answer is self-explanatory.

18. Acid production within dental plaque reaches demineralizing concentrations after ingestion of carbohydrates within:

(*a*) 4 minutes (*b*) 15 minutes

(*c*) 30 minutes (*d*) 25 minutes

Answer (*a*).

The answer is self-explanatory.

19. Which of the following is the mechanism by which fluoride exerts the cariostatic action?

(*a*) Incorporation of fluoride into dentin and enamel of unerupted teeth.

(*b*) Secretion of fluoride in saliva, which decreases acid production in plaque and enhances remineralization of enamel.

(*c*) Fluoride in saliva helps in maturation of enamel of newly erupted teeth which decreases caries susceptibility.

(*d*) All of the above.

Answer (*d*).

All the above mentioned factors are true regarding cariostatic action of fluoride.

20. The most effective method of reducing the incidence of caries in the general population is:

(*a*) school water fluoridation

(*b*) community water fluoridation

(*c*) fluoridated tooth paste

(*d*) salt fluoridation

Answer (*b*).

Community water fluoridation has proved to be the best method for reducing the incidence of caries in general population.

21. The first fluoride containing dentifrice (CREST) had:

(*a*) stannous fluoride

(*b*) sodium fluoride

(*c*) acidulated phosphate fluoride

(*d*) sodium mono-fluorophosphate

Answer (*a*).

The dentifrice CREST contained stannous fluoride in combination with calcium pyrophosphate as the cleaning and polishing system and was accepted as the first therapeutic dentifrice by the council on dental therapeutics of the American Dental Association in 1964.

22. The concentration of sodium fluoride used for professional topical fluoride application is:

(*a*) 0.2% (*b*) 2%

(*c*) 0.02% (*d*) 0.002%

Answer (*b*).

Four applications of 2% sodium fluoride solution during a 2- week period, with the series of applications at 2–3 year intervals has shown to decrease the caries incidence by 40%.

23. The concentration of stannous fluoride and acidulated phosphate fluoride used for professional topical fluoride application are:

(*a*) 8% and 12.3% (*b*) 0.8% and 1.23%

(*c*) 0.8% and 12.3% (*d*) 8% and 1.23%

Answer (*d*).

Stannous fluoride is available in powder form, in either bulk containers or pre-weighed capsules. The recommended concentration is 8%. Acidulated phosphate fluoride (APF-1.23%) is available as either a solution, a gel or a foam all of which are stable and ready to use.

24. All of the following are true regarding stannous fluoride except:

(*a*) 8% stannous fluoride solution is obtained by dissolving 0.8 gms of powder in 100 ml of distilled water

(*b*) Stannous fluoride solutions are acidic with a pH of 2.4–2.8

(*c*) Stannous fluoride solution is not stable, hence it has to be prepared immediately before use

(*d*) Stannous fluoride is available in powder form in either bulk containers or pre-weighed capsules

Answer (*a*).

Stannous fluoride (8%) is obtained by dissolving 0.8 g of powder in 10 ml of distilled water.

25. APF gel or solution contains all except:

(*a*) sodium fluoride (*b*) hydrofluoric acid

(*c*) phosphoric acid (*d*) hydrochloric acid

Answer (*d*).

APF system consists essentially of mixture of sodium fluoride, hydrofluoric acid, and phosphoric acid, with concentrations of 1.23% fluoride and 0.98% phosphoric acid with a pH of 3 to 3.5.

26. APF gels can be usually stored for:

(*a*) 1 year (*b*) 2 years

(*c*) 5 years (*d*) 4.5 years

Answer (*b*).

The APF systems are chemically stable for at least 2 years when stored in plastic containers, but there may be a decrease in the viscosity of the gels after several months of storage.

27. The usual time recommended for topical fluoride application is:

(*a*) 4 minutes (*b*) 8 minutes

(*c*) 2 minutes (*d*) 6 minutes

Answer (*a*).

A 4-minute treatment time is recommended for either solution or gel. Topical application of APF gel, solution or foam should be repeated at least every 6 months.

28. Which of the following is/are true about carrying out a topical fluoride application for a child patient?

(*a*) Both trays can be inserted at once.

(*b*) Patient sits in a upright position with head tipped slightly forward to allow excess saliva and gel to flow towards the lips.

(*c*) The trays are in place for 4 minutes.

(*d*) Patient may need assistance or positive reinforcement during the procedure.

(*e*) All of the above.

Answer (*e*).

The choices describe the technique of application.

29. Patients are encouraged not to drink, eat, or rinse after fluoride application for:

(*a*) 1 hour

(*b*) 15 minutes

(*c*) 30 minutes

(*d*) 90 minutes

Answer (*c*).

Patients are encouraged not to drink, eat, or rinse after fluoride application for thirty minutes to maximize the fluoride uptake into the enamel.

30. The concentration of fluoride used for mouth rinse is:

(*a*) 0.2% NaF rinse once weekly

(*b*) 0.05% NaF rinse once daily

(*c*) both a and b

(*d*) 0.02% NaF rinse once daily and 0.05% NaF rinse once weekly

Answer (*c*).

The answer is self-explanatory.

31. Transfer of fluoride does occur from the mother to the foetus through placenta. The benefit of caries prevention is more for the primary teeth than the permanent teeth because of this transmission from mother to foetus.

(*a*) Both the statements are false.

(*b*) Both the statements are true.

(*c*) First statement is true and the second is false.

(*d*) First statement is false and the second is true.

Answer (*b*).

Transfer of fluorides does occur from mother to foetus. Those who support prenatal fluorides usage agreed to this point. However, how much fluoride is transferred from the mother's blood remains uncertain. Researchers generally agree that some benefits accrue to the primary teeth but considerable doubt exists about the benefits to the permanent teeth.

32. The administration of fluoride supplements should commence shortly after birth and should continue through the time of eruption of second permanent

molars. If the natural fluoride content of water is 0.7 ppm or more supplements should not be recommended.

(*a*) Both the statements are false.

(*b*) Both the statements are true.

(*c*) First statement is true and the second is false.

(*d*) First statement is false and the second is true.

Answer (*b*).

The answer is self-explanatory.

33. One of the following is not a disadvantage of stannous fluoride topical application:

(*a*) bad taste

(*b*) etch porcelain restoration

(*c*) stain silicate restoration

(*d*) pigmentation of arrested lesions

Answer (*b*).

Stannous fluoride solutions do not etch porcelain restorations like APF gels or solutions. Hence, this is an advantage of stannous fluoride solutions.

34. All of the following are advantages of APF gel except:

(*a*) it has a better taste than stannous fluoride

(*b*) it has no staining or pigmentation

(*c*) it can be applied to both arches simultaneously

(*d*) it does not damage porcelain restorations

Answer (*d*).

Refer to the explanation of Q. No. 33.

35. The quantity of stannous fluoride solution required for treating a patient is approximately:

(*a*) 10 ml (*b*) 20 ml

(*c*) 30 ml (*d*) 40 ml

Answer (*a*).

The answer is self-explanatory.

36. In tray application of APF gel, the quantity of gel taken for one application is:

(*a*) 2/3 of the trough area of the tray

(*b*) 1/3 of the trough area of the tray

(*c*) fill the tray completely

(*d*) less than 1/3 of the trough area of the tray

Answer (*b*).

APF gel or foam is placed to fill one-third of the trough area so that it fits properly over each dental arch. Avoid overloading the tray, this could lead to excessive ingestion.

37. Sodium fluoride solution is a:

(*a*) neutral solution

(*b*) acidic solution

(*c*) alkaline solution

(*d*) none of the above

Answer (*a*).

Sodium fluoride solutions are of neutral pH and have a more acceptable taste than stannous fluoride.

38. The fluoridated dentifrice has fluoride in the following concentration:

(*a*) 1000–1100 ppm

(*b*) 200–300 ppm

(*c*) 2000–2500 ppm

(*d*) 1800–2200 ppm

Answer (*a*).

The answer is self-explanatory. A 25% to 35% caries reduction can be expected with the use of fluoride dentifrices. Increased benefit is observed with two or three brushings per day when compared to one brushing.

39. Gel-Kam has:

(*a*) 0.4% NaF

(*b*) 0.4% APF

(*c*) 0.4% Stannous fluoride

(*d*) 0.6% NaF

Answer (*c*).

Gel-Kam has 0.4% stannous fluoride (1000 ppm F).

40. The fluoride concentration in school water fluoridation is:

(*a*) 2 times the city water supply

(*b*) 4.5 times the city water supply

(*c*) 8 times the city water supply

(*d*) equal as the city water supply

Answer (*b*).

The answer is self-explanatory. School-water fluoridation shows 35% caries reduction with supervised daily or weekly rinses.

41. Communal water fluoridation is the most effective method of caries prevention in general population. Optimal concentration of fluoride in community-water fluoridation varies with mean annual area temperature.

(*a*) Both the statements are false.

(*b*) Both the statements are true.

(*c*) First statement is true and the second is false.

(*d*) First statement is false and the second is true.

Answer (*b*).

Optimal concentration varies with the mean annual temperature because of the varied water consumption in different temperatures. If the mean temperature of a particular area is high then the optimal fluoride concentration is kept less in that area.

42. Which of the following properties of saliva have been investigated for their role in caries process?

(*a*) Salivary pH.

(*b*) Buffering capacity of saliva or acid neutralizing power of saliva.

(*c*) Calcium and phosphorous content of saliva.

(*d*) All of the above.

Answer (*d*).

The answer is self-explanatory. Other properties like flow rate, viscosity and bacteriostatic and bactericidal substances of saliva have also been investigated for their role in caries process.

43. Match the following:

S. No.	*Gland*	*S. No.*	*Type of secretion*
1.	Submaxillary	A	Thin watery and low in organic content.
2.	Sublingual	B	Mixed type of fluid—a thin watery type and a thick viscid juice rich in mucin.
3.	Parotid	C	Predominantly mucous, few serous alveoli. Secretion may be thin and watery or viscid, depending on the nature of the secretory stimulus. It is usually mucous.

(*a*) 1-A, 2-B, 3-C (*b*) 1-B, 2-C, 3-A

(*c*) 1-C, 2-A, 3-B Answer (*b*).

The answer is self-explanatory.

Gland-stimulus secretion

S. No.	*Gland*	*Parasympathetic*	*Sympathetic*
1.	Submaxillary	Profuse watery secretion	Scanty thick mucinous juice
2.	Sublingual	Profuse watery secretion	Scanty thick mucinous juice
3.	Parotid	Profuse watery secretion	No secretion

44. The first report of a severe salivary deficiency with its deleterious effect on the dentition was reported by:

(*a*) Hutchinson in 1888

(*b*) Keyes in 1910

(*c*) Jenson in 1890

(*d*) Snyder in 1915

Answer (*a*).

The answer is self-explanatory.

45. Which of the following conditions is associated with dry mouth or salivary gland dysfunction?

(*a*) Use of anti-histamine drugs

(*b*) Use of chlorpromazine

(*c*) Myasthenia gravis

(*d*) All of the above

Answer (*d*).

Often the first symptom of salivary deficiency is the rapid deterioration of teeth. Acquired salivary deficiency may be the result of a psychic or emotional disturbances and may be either temporary or permanent in nature. Immune disorders such as Sjogren syndrome and ectodermal dysplasia often exhibit xerostomia.

46. To evaluate salivary flow, saliva should be collected at least ____________ after a meal:

(*a*) 90 minutes (*b*) 3 hours

(*c*) 30 minutes (*d*) 4 hours

Answer (*a*).

Although there is little daily or seasonal variation in a person's salivary flow, the saliva should be collected at the same time each day (for example at least 11/2 hours after a meal).

47. Salivary flow increases 0.78 ml each year up to 35 years of age. Estimated stimulated salivary flow of the infant is 5.6 ml for 15 minutes.

(*a*) Both the statements are false.

(*b*) Both the statements are true.

(*c*) First statement is true and the second is false.

(*d*) First statement is false and the second is true.

Answer (*b*).

The normal stimulated flow for persons of different ages can be calculated with the following equation: 0.78 X Age + 5.6* = stimulated flow/15 minutes.

48. The lactobacillus count test to assess caries activity was introduced by:

(*a*) Hadley 1933 (*b*) Jay 1933

(*c*) Snyder (*d*) Edelstein

Answer (*a*).

The lactobacillus count test was introduced by Hadley in 1933 and popularized by Jay. At present this test is limited to research studies.

49. Alban test is a simplified substitute for the Snyder test. These tests are designed for a quantitative determination of the number of acid-producing organisms in saliva.

(*a*) Both the statements are false.

(*b*) Both the statements are true.

(*c*) First statement is true and the second is false.

(*d*) First statement is false and the second is true.

Answer (*b*).

Snyder introduced a colorimetric test for the estimation of relative numbers of lactobacilli in saliva. Later this was modified by Alban. This test quantitatively determines the acid-producing microorganisms in saliva. These tests were once widely used as diagnostic tools to evaluate patient's acceptance of dietary changes and preventive measures designed to reduce dental caries.

50. Caries risk test was given by:

(*a*) Hadley 1933

(*b*) Jay 1933

(*c*) Snyder

(*d*) Edelstein and Tinanoff

Answer (*d*).

The caries risk test described by Edelstein and Tinanoff and by Weinberger and Wright were initially expected to be useful to the dentist who seeks to distinguish the caries competent and caries incompetent child, both of whom appear caries free on examination. However the practicality and accuracy of such tests have not proved as helpful as anticipated.

51. Moisten a sterile tongue blade with unstimulated saliva and then impress it onto the raised surface of a Mitis salivarius medium in Rodac plates. After the incubation, examine the plates for Streptococus mutans colonies. This test is known as:

(*a*) Snyder test

(*b*) Alban test

(*c*) Caries risk test

(*d*) Modified Lactobacillus test

Answer (*c*).

Refer to the explanation of Q. No. 50.

52. Which of the following caries activity tests were widely used as diagnostic tools and to evaluate patients

acceptance of dietary changes and preventive measures designed to reduce dental caries?

(*a*) Snyder test

(*b*) Alban test

(*c*) Caries risk test

(*d*) Both (*a*) and (*b*)

Answer (*d*).

Refer to the explanation of Q. No. 49.

Chapter 8

Oral Hygiene Measures

1. The length of bristles in most of the toothbrushes is:

(*a*) 5–8 mm (*b*) 11 mm

(*c*) 15 mm (*d*) 18 mm

Answer (*b*).

The length of bristles in most of the toothbrushes is 11 mm. Brushes are classified as soft, medium or hard based on the width of the bristles. The diameter ranges from 0.16 to 0.22 mm for soft, 0.23 to 0.29 mm for medium and 0.30 mm and greater for hard toothbrushes.

2. Which of the following bristle ends cause the least amount of gingival irritation?

(*a*) Coarse cut (*b*) Enlarged bulbous

(*c*) Round end (*d*) None of the above

Answer (*c*).

The three types of bristle ends are coarse cut, enlarged bulbous and round end. Of the three types of bristle ends the round end is the bristle-type of choice because of its decreased incidence of gingival tissue irritation. However even the coarse-cut bristles round off eventually with normal use.

3. Which of the following is true regarding the powered toothbrush—Interplak?

(*a*) It uses the movement of individual tufts of bristles rather than the head of the brush.

(*b*) Interplak has 10 independently driven tufts that rotate approximately 4200 times per minute.

(*c*) Each soft bristled tuft alternatively rotates 11/2 revolutions in one direction and then reverses to rotate 11/2 revolutions in the opposite direction with adjacent tufts rotating in opposite direction.

(*d*) All of the above.

Answer (*d*).

All the above-mentioned facts are true regarding the powered tooth brush—Interplak.

4. The novelty of the powered toothbrushes causes an initial increase in use and therefore control of plaque and gingivitis. Any change or experimental manipulation similar to the above situation may induce an improvement in behaviour, which is known as the Hawthorne effect?

(*a*) Both the statements are false.

(*b*) Both the statements are true.

(*c*) First statement is true and the second is false.

(*d*) First statement is false and the second is true.

Answer (*b*).

A few studies have confirmed that powered toothbrushes are not as effective as manual brushes in plaque removal for a typical patient over a protracted period. Kerlinger attributes the initial increase in use and initial improvement in plaque and gingivitis control to the novelty of the powered toothbrush. Over time the results become comparable to manual brushing.

5. The soft brush is preferable for most uses in pediatric dentistry because of:

(*a*) decreased incidence of gingival tissue trauma

(*b*) increased interproximal cleaning ability

(*c*) the bristle type is usually round end

(*d*) all of the above

Answer (*d*).

The answer is self-explanatory.

6. The advantage of the new floss made up of Teflon material is:

(*a*) it has lower coefficient of friction than nylon

(*b*) it slides easily between tight contacts and minimizes snapping of the floss

(*c*) it does not shred

(*d*) all of the above

Answer (*d*).

Several different types of floss are available—flavoured and unflavoured; waxed and unwaxed; thin, tape and meshwork. Almost all commercially available floss is made up of nylon. The newly introduced floss made up of Teflon material has the above advantages.

7. Which of the following dye is used in disclosing agents?

(*a*) Gentian violet (*b*) Erythrosin

(*c*) Fluorescein (*d*) Basic fuchsin

(*e*) Any of the above

Answer (*e*).

Disclosing agents include iodine, gentian violet, erythrosin, basic fuchsin, fast green, food dyes, fluorescein, etc.

8. The brushing technique naturally adopted by children is:

(*a*) rolling stroke method

(*b*) Horizontal scrub method

(*c*) Charters' method

(*d*) modified Stillman method

Answer (*b*).

The horizontal scrub technique removes as much plaque or more plaque than other techniques, regardless of the child's age or if the parent performs the brushing. In addition, it is the technique most naturally adopted by children.

9. Lap-to-lap position is a recommended position for performing oral hygiene procedures in:

(*a*) infants (0–1 year old)

(*b*) toddlers (1–3 years old)

(*c*) preschool child (3–6 years old)

(*d*) school age (6–12 years old)

Answer (*b*).

Two adults sit with knees touching using their laps as a table to rest the child. One adult holds the child's legs and arms while the other adult performs the oral hygiene procedures.

10. The oldest antiplaque agent is:

(*a*) Listerine

(*b*) Chlorhexidine

(*c*) cetylpyridinium chloride

(*d*) sanguinarine

Answer (*a*).

The most widely known non-charged phenolic antiseptic agent is Listerine. It has demonstrated a long history of efficacy and was among the original antiseptic agents studied by W.D. Miller in 1890.

11. Dentrifices:

(*a*) act as plaque and stain-removing agents

(*b*) have pleasant colours and flavours which encourage their use

(*c*) have tartar control properties

(*d*) have anticaries and desensitizing properties

(*e*) all the statements are true

Answer (*e*).

Dentrifices serve multiple functions in oral hygiene through the use of a variety of agents. They act as plaque and stain-removing agents through the use of abrasives and surfactants. They have tartar control properties with the addition of pyrophosphates. They have anticaries and desensitization properties through the action of fluoride and other agents.

12. All the following statements are true except:

(*a*) more time was spent brushing the upper than lower teeth by the children

(*b*) the contralateral side was brushed more than the ipsilateral side in children (*c*) less than 10% of the time was spent in brushing the lingual areas

(*d*) most popular brushing stroke was the horizontal scrub method in children

Answer (*a*).

The answer is self-explanatory.

13. Which of the following mouth rinse has the highest alcohol content?

(*a*) Listerine

(*b*) Chlorhexidine

(*c*) Cetylpyridinium chloride

(*d*) Sanguinarine

Answer (*a*).

In mouthwashes, Listerine has one of the highest alcohol content approximately 25%.

14. The usual concentration of chlorhexidine used for mouth rinsing is:

(*a*) 0.2% (*b*) 0.02%

(*c*) 0.002% (*d*) 2%

Answer (*a*).

The answer is self-explanatory.

15. Disclosing agents are available in all of the following forms except:

(*a*) tablets (*b*) wafers

(*c*) gels (*d*) capsules

Answer (*c*).

Disclosing gels are not available. These agents are highly desirable for effective plaque removal and patient motivation. A good disclosing agent stains the teeth only very faintly by staining the pellicle a faint pink colour but stains the dental plaque deeply and vividly.

16. The first commercial dental floss was probably introduced in:

(*a*) 1782 (*b*) 1882

(*c*) 1970 (*d*) 1910

Answer (*b*).

The first commercial dental floss was introduced in 1882 in Massachusetts and the first patent on dental floss dates back to 1876. The Johnson and Johnson Company manufactured silk dental flosses as early as 1898.

17. All of the following about dental floss is/are true except:

(*a*) no difference in effectiveness of plaque removal exists between waxed and unwaxed floss

(*b*) waxed floss tends to fray more than unwaxed floss

(*c*) each dental floss depending on its thickness is made with 4–18 ends of filaments twisted in a predetermined number of twists per inch.

(*d*) waxed floss is used much more in dental offices than unwaxed floss

Answer (*b*).

Bass was a strong proponent of the unwaxed floss because of fear of wax being left on the interproximal surfaces from waxed floss and also unwaxed floss is usually thinner and splays more on use.

18. Which of the following is/are undesirable side-effects of chlorhexidine?

(*a*) Brown diffuse discolouration of teeth.

(*b*) Unpleasant bitter taste.

(*c*) Dryness of the mouth.

(*d*) Burning sensations of the tongue.

(*e*) All of the above.

Answer (*e*).

The answer is self-explanatory.

19. An ideal chemotherapeutic plaque control agent should have:

(*a*) specificity only for pathogenic bacteria

(*b*) substantivity and chemical stability

(*c*) toxicologic and ecologic safety

(*d*) ease of use

(*e*) all of the above

Answer (*e*).

Substantivity is the ability to attach to and be retained by oral surfaces and then be released overtime without loss of potency. Though no agent has yet been developed that has all the above features, chemotherapeutic agents still play a role in maintaining oral health.

Chapter 9

Pit and Fissure Sealants

1. The concentration of phosphoric acid used for acid etching usually is:

(*a*) 30–50% acid solution or gel

(*b*) 10–20% acid solution

(*c*) 70–80% acid solution or gel

(*d*) less than 10%

Answer (*a*).

The answer is self-explanatory.

2. Generally a 20 second etching time is recommended. Enamel that has been exposed to fluoride may be resistant to etching and may need to be exposed for longer periods.

(*a*) Both the statements are false.

(*b*) Both the statements are true.

(*c*) First statement is true and the second is false.

(*d*) First statement is false and the second is true.

Answer (b).

The answer is self-explanatory.

3. Which of the following are advantages of light-cured materials over chemical-cure sealants?

(*a*) Less chance of incorporation of air bubbles.
(*b*) Working time is longer.
(*c*) Better physical and mechanical properties.
(*d*) All of the above.

Answer (d).

All of the above mentioned factors are true regarding light-cure materials.

4. The sealed composite resin restoration (preve ntive resin restoration) is an alternative procedure to restore young permanent teeth that require only minimal tooth preparation for caries removal but also have adjacent susceptible fissures. This conservative cavity preparation with sealing for prevention is a successful approach for treating selected decayed teeth.

(*a*) Both the statements are false.
(*b*) Both the statements are true.
(*c*) First statement is true and the second is false.
(*d*) First statement is false and the second is true.

Answer (b).

The answer is self-explanatory.

5. Acid etching was introduced by:

(*a*) Bowen (1965)

(*b*) Buonocore (1955)

(*c*) Wilson and Kent (1972)

(*d*) Brown (1945)

Answer (*b*).

Bowen introduced the Bis-GMA resin system. Buonocore introduced acid etching. Wilson and Kent introduced Glass Ionomer cement.

6. Bis-GMA resin was developed by:

(*a*) Bowen (1965)

(*b*) Buonocore (1955)

(*c*) Wilson and Kent (1972)

(*d*) Brown (1945)

Answer (*a*).

Refer to the explanation of Q. No. 5.

Bis-GMA resin is the chemical reation product of Bisphenol A and Glycidyl methacrylate. It is the base resin to most of the current commercial sealants.

7. Match the following:

	Resin		***Activator***
A	Chemically curing resins	1.	Benzoin methyl ether
B	U-V curing resins	2.	Diketones
C	Visible light curing resins	3.	Tertiary amines

(*a*) A-3, B-1, C-2 (*b*) A-2, B-3, C-1

(*c*) A-1, B-2, C-3

Answer (*a*).

The answer is self-explanatory.

Chapter 10

Pediatric Operative Dentistry

1. Use of rubber dam offers the following advantages:

(*a*) saves time

(*b*) provides protection

(*c*) controls saliva

(*d*) all of the above

Answer (*d*).

The time required for application of rubber dam ranges from 15 seconds to 6 minutes. This time required for the placement will be invariably made up and additional time saved through the elimination of rinsing and spitting by the pediatric patient. It prevents foreign objects from coming into contact with oral structures. It also prevents swallowing or aspiration of foreign objects and materials. Rubber dam effectively controls the saliva, helping the operator to identify small pulp exposures easily and place restorative materials on the tooth without contamination.

2. The latex sheets used for rubber dam is usually of ____________ size.

(*a*) 5 × 5 inch

(*b*) 2 × 2 inch

(*c*) 1 × 1 inch

(*d*) 6 × 6 inch

Answer (*a*).

The armamentarium of rubber dam consists usually 5 × 5 inch latex sheets. Smaller sheets are available for pediatric patients.

3. The framework used for rubber dam application is otherwise called:

(*a*) Clark's frame

(*b*) Young's frame

(*c*) Barnum's frame

(*d*) Nicholos frame

Answer (*b*).

The answer is self-explanatory.

4. The smallest punch hole created by rubber dam punch is used to isolate:

(*a*) mandibular premolars

(*b*) primary incisors

(*c*) mandibular permanent incisors

(*d*) both (*b*) and (*c*)

Answer (*d*).

The large punch hole is used for the clamp-bearing tooth and for the most permanent molars. The medium-sized punch holes are generally used for the premolars and primary molars. The second smallest hole is used for maxillary permanent incisors, whereas the smallest hole is adequate for the primary incisors and the lower permanent incisors.

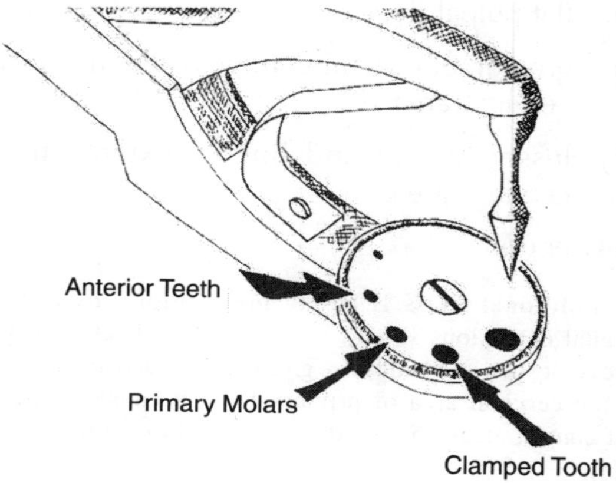

Fig. 10.1 Rubber dam punch.

5. Rounded angles throughout the cavity preparation (Class II) will result in:

(*a*) less concentration of stresses

(*b*) complete condensation of amalgam (more bulk)

(*c*) both (*a*) and (*b*)

(*d*) prevention of thermal stimulus injuring the pulp

Answer (*c*).

Rounded angle throughout the cavity preparation will result in less concentration of stresses and will permit better adaptation of the materials into the extremities of the preparation.

6. All of the following are true regarding Class II cavity preparation in primary molars except:

(*a*) buccal and lingual extension carried to self cleansing areas (*b*) flat pulpal floor

(*c*) greater buccal and lingual extension at the cervical area

(*d*) lesser buccal and lingual extension at the cervical area

Answer (*d*).

In traditional Class II cavity preparation, the buccal and lingual extensions should be carried to self-cleansing areas. The cavity design should have greater buccal and lingual extension in the cervical area of primary teeth because of the broad, flat contact areas and the distinct buccal bulge in the gingival third.

7. Ideally the width of the isthmus should be:

(*a*) half the intercuspal distance

(*b*) one-third the intercuspal distance

(*c*) one-fourth the intercuspal distance

(*d*) three-fourth the intercuspal distance

Answer (*b*).

The strength at the isthmus area of a Class II cavity is three times greater when the bulk of amalgam alloy is provided in depth rather than in width. The recommended width in primary teeth is one-third of the intercuspal distance.

8. During cavity preparation the floor of the cavity is extended into dentinoenamel junction by:

(*a*) 0.05 mm (*b*) 0.5 mm

(*c*) 5 mm (*d*) 0.2 mm

Answer (*b*).

Limiting the cavity to 0.5 mm pulpal to dentinoenamel junction reduces the chance of inadvertent pulp exposure.

9. All of the following are true regarding Class I cavity preparation except:

(*a*) preparation includes all susceptible grooves and fissures

(*b*) depth of the cavity is carried to 0.5 mm below DE junction

(*c*) undermining marginal ridges strengthen the tooth

(*d*) all unsupported enamel rods are removed

Answer (*c*).

If the marginal ridges are undermined the enamel is more susceptible to fracture.

10. A Class II cavity preparation comprises:

(*a*) occlusal preparation

(*b*) proximal box

(*c*) isthmus

(*d*) all of the above

Answer (*d*).

The answer is self-explanatory.

11. The buccal and lingual walls of the proximal box in a Class II preparation should:

(*a*) diverge towards the cervical region

(*b*) converge towards the cervical region

(*c*) diverge towards the occlusal region

(*d*) none of the above

Answer (*a*).

Refer to the explanation of Q. No. 6.

12. The most common cause for failure of an amalgam restoration is:

(*a*) proximal ditch

(*b*) delayed expansion

(*c*) failure at occlusal preparation

(*d*) due to poor handling of amalgam alloy

Answer (*a*).

Breakdown of the material in the proximal wall region results in a defect known as proximal ditch. This leads to marginal leakage and secondary caries resulting in failure of the restoration.

13. A MOD amalgam has a better survival rate in:

(*a*) mandibular second primary molar than first primary molar

(*b*) mandibular first primary molar than second primary molar

(*c*) all primary molars

(*d*) none of the above

Answer (*a*).

A MOD has a better survival rate in mandibular second primary molars. However, multisurface decay is better managed by the placement of a stainless steel crown.

14. One of the following is incorrectly defined:

(*a*) Class I—preparation involving pits and fissures in posterior teeth

(*b*) Class II—preparation involving occlusal and proximal surfaces

(*c*) Class III—preparation in proximal surfaces of anteriors involving the incisal edge

(*d*) Class V—preparation in the cervical region of teeth

Answer (*c*).

Class III is preparation without involving the incisal edge. Preparation involving the incisal edge is classified as Class IV.

15. The modified Class III preparation uses a dovetail on the lingual side in:

(*a*) maxillary canine

(*b*) mandibular canine

(*c*) mandibular premolar

(*d*) maxillary premolar

Answer (*a*).

The modified Class III preparation uses a dovetail on the lingual or occasionally on the labial surfaces of the tooth. A lingual lock is normally considered for the maxillary canine, whereas the labial lock may be more conveniently cut on the mandibular teeth where the esthetic requirement is not so important.

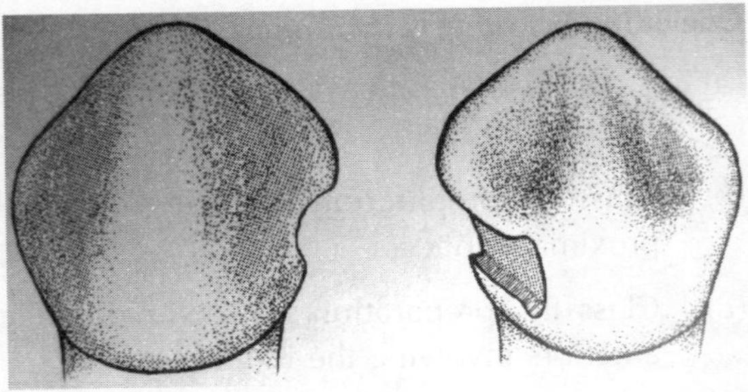

Fig. 10.2 Class III in mandibular canine—Labial dovetail (lingual and labial views).

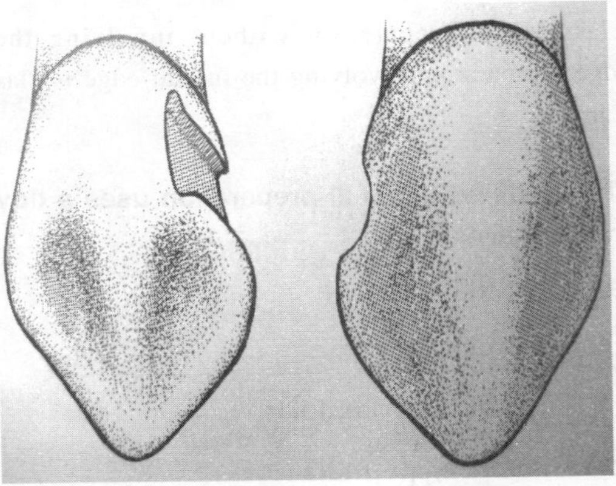

Fig. 10.3 Class III in maxillary canine—Lingual dovetail (lingual and labial views).

16. In a Class II preparation in permanent first molar, retention of the proximal box:

(*a*) depends on retention of the occlusal preparation

(*b*) is independent of the occlusal preparation
(*c*) is not necessary
(*d*) is because of the occlusal divergence of the box

Answer (*b*).

Retention of the restoration results from the mechanical undercut obtained by the extension into the fissures of the occlusal part and the diverging walls of the proximal box. It is important that retention of the interproximal box and the occlusal part are independent of each other, as they may be subjected to different displacement forces.

17. Outline of the cavity for amalgam restoration is determined by:

(*a*) size of the carious lesion
(*b*) the need for extension for prevention
(*c*) occlusal anatomy of the tooth
(*d*) all of the above

Answer (*d*).

All the above mentioned factors have to be considered while determining the outline form for cavity preparation.

18. The most commonly used base in deep cavities after removal of deep caries is:

(*a*) calcium hydroxide powder
(*b*) hard setting calcium hydroxide
(*c*) zinc oxide eugenol
(*d*) polycarboxylate cement

Answer (*b*).

With deep carious lesions and near-pulp exposures, the depth of the cavity should be covered with a biocompatible base material to provide adequate thermal protection to the pulp. A hard setting calcium hydroxide is generally used for this purpose.

19. The primary purpose of applying cavity varnish is to prevent:

(*a*) thermal damage to the pulp

(*b*) marginal leakage

(*c*) discoloration of tooth

(*d*) pulp exposure

Answer (*b*).

Cavity varnishes are used to prevent marginal leakage and bases are used to provide thermal protection to the pulp.

20. Preservation of primary dentition will always prevent a malocclusion. Early loss of primary molars causes more severe effects than early loss of primary incisors.

(*a*) First statement is false and the second is true.

(*b*) First statement is true and the second is false.

(*c*) Both the statements are true.

(*d*) Both the statements are false.

Answer (*a*).

Preservation of primary dentition prevents malocclusion but not always. Early loss of primary incisors does not usually cause space loss.

21. Which of the following is true of chemicoparasitic theory of dental caries?

(*a*) Introduced by Miller (1890).

(*b*) Otherwise called acidogenic theory.

(*c*) Streptococci mutans and lactobacilli are the probable causative microorganisms.

(*d*) All of the above.

Answer (*d*).

According to Miller, the above mentioned acidogenic microorganisms utilize the refined carbohydrates and produce acids, which dissolve the enamel resulting in a cavity.

22. Recommended age for discontinuing bottle-feeding is:

(*a*) 12 months (*b*) 8 months

(*c*) 20 months (*d*) 18 months

Answer (*a*).

Prolongation of bottle-feeding beyond 12 months of age can result in early childhood caries.

23. Early childhood caries can occur because of:

(*a*) prolonged bottle-feeding

(*b*) at will breast-feeding

(*c*) frequent use of sweetened syrupy medicines

(*d*) any of the above

Answer (*d*).

All of the above mentioned factors create a susceptible environment in the mouth by the presence of sucrose around the tooth, which results in early childhood caries.

24. Nursing caries affects primarily the lingual surfaces of primary maxillary incisors and occlusal surfaces of

first primary molars. The mandibular incisors are characteristically unaffected.

(*a*) Both the statements are true.

(*b*) Both the statements are false.

(*c*) First statement is true and the second is false.

(*d*) First statement is false and the second is true.

Answer (*a*).

The answer is self-explanatory.

25. All of the following are true regarding rampant caries except:

(*a*) a rapidly spreading burrowing type of caries

(*b*) early involvement of pulp

(*c*) usually affects teenagers and young adolescents

(*d*) affect teeth usually not immune to tooth decay

Answer (*d*).

Massler has defined rampant caries as a rapidly spreading, burrowing type of caries, which show early pulp involvement and affect teeth, which are usually immune to tooth decay.

26. Enamel rods in the gingival one-third of primary teeth incline:

(*a*) horizontally (*b*) occlusally

(*c*) apically (*d*) gingivally

Answer (*b*).

Enamel rods incline occlusally in primary teeth in the cervical region; hence, beveling of gingival seat is not required in Class II cavity preparations. However, in permanent teeth they incline gingivally. When a gingival seat is prepared in this region it results in unsupported enamel, which requires beveling.

27. All of the following are true regarding contact areas in primary teeth except:

(*a*) broad contact area

(*b*) flatter contact area

(*c*) situated more occlusally

(*d*) need to be broken in Class II cavity preparation

Answer (*c*).

The contact areas between the primary molars are broader, flatter and situated farther gingivally than those between the permanent molars.

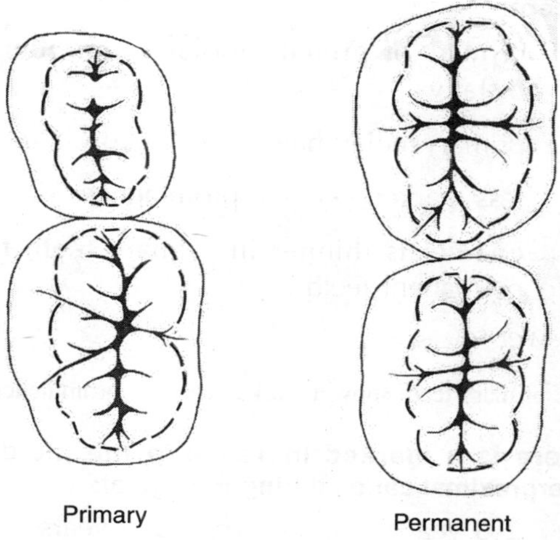

Fig. 10.4 Picture depicting broad contact areas in primary teeth.

28. The pulp horns of primary teeth are less prominent and relatively far from the surface. The distobuccal pulp horn of mandibular first primary molar is exposed often during restorative procedures.

(*a*) Both the statements are true.

(*b*) Both the statements are false.

(*c*) First statement is true and the second is false.

(*d*) First statement is false and the second is true.

Answer (*b*).

The reverse is true. The pulp horns of primary teeth are more prominent than those of permanent teeth and are relatively closer to the surface when the thinner primary enamel is considered. The mesiobuccal pulp horn of mandibular first primary molar is exposed often during restorative procedures.

29. All of the following are true regarding primary teeth except:

(*a*) crowns of primary molars are wider mesio-distally

(*b*) primary molars have a very narrow occlusal table

(*c*) less marked cervical prominence

(*d*) enamel is thinner in primary teeth than the permanent teeth

Answer (*c*).

The primary teeth show a marked cervical prominence.

30. There is a marked increase in the incidence of interproximal caries during the age of:

(*a*) 2–3 years (*b*) 3–5 years

(*c*) 7–9 years (*d*) 6–8 years

Answer (*b*).

Occlusal lesions are more common than interproximal lesions in preschool children. In these young children posterior contact may not close until the age of 3, which may explain this observation. Once the proximal contacts are established, the incidence of interproximal caries starts increasing.

31. Whenever possible, facial and lingual walls of the proximal box of a Class II cavity in the primary molar should be:

(*a*) flared as much as possible

(*b*) rounded as much as possible

(*c*) kept as parallel as possible

(*d*) parallel to the respective external surfaces of tooth

Answer (*d*).

The facial and lingual walls of the proximal box of a Class II cavity in the primary molar should be parallel to the respective external surfaces of the tooth.

32. In which of the primary molars does the anatomy of the pulp contraindicate an MOD preparation for the placement of an amalgam restoration:

(*a*) maxillary first molar

(*b*) maxillary second molar

(*c*) mandibular first molar

(*d*) mandibular second molar

Answer (*c*).

Mandibular first primary molar has a prominent cervical bulge, which makes it a poor candidate for MOD preparation.

Chapter 11

Pulp Therapy

1. A tooth that has been treated successfully with a pulpotomy technique should have after one year:

(*a*) a normal periodontal ligament and lamina dura

(*b*) radiographic evidence of a calcified bridge if calcium hydroxide had been used as a capping material

(*c*) no radiographic evidence of internal resorption

(*d*) all of the above

Answer (*d*).

All of the above mentioned factors are true regarding the success of a pulpotomized tooth.

2. A patient aged 7 years complains of severe toothache at night in relation to 75. The mode of treatment probably will be:

(*a*) pulpotomy

(*b*) pulpectomy

(*c*) direct pulp capping

(*d*) indirect pulp capping

Answer (*b*).

Nocturnal pain indicates irreversible pulpitis. Hence the treatment options can be pulpectomy or extraction. The nocturnal pain associated with the tooth increases in the night because of the patient's posture which increases the blood flow to the head and neck. This in turn increases the intrapulpal pressure, which results in severe toothache.

3. A severe toothache at night usually means extensive degeneration of the pulp. This calls for more than a conservative type of pulp therapy.

(*a*) Both the statements are false.

(*b*) Both the statements are true.

(*c*) First statement is true and the second is false.

(*d*) First statement is false and the second is true.

Answer (*b*).

The answer is self-explanatory.

Refer to the explanation of Q. No. 2.

4. All of the following statements are true regarding gingival abscess except:

(*a*) a gingival abscess or draining fistula associated with deep carious lesion is an obvious clinical sign of irreversibly diseased pulp

(*b*) such infections can be resolved only by successful endodontic therapy or extraction of the tooth

(*c*) gingival abscess is also known as parulis

(*d*) a gingival abscess or a draining fistula associated with a tooth with a deep carious lesion is an obvious clinical sign of reversibly diseased pulp

Answer (*d*).

The answer is self-explanatory.

5. A gingival abscess or a draining fistula associated with a tooth with a deep carious lesion is an obvious clinical sign of:

(*a*) reversibly diseased pulp

(*b*) irreversibly diseased pulp

(*c*) beginning of pulpal degeneration

(*d*) healthy radicular pulp and infected coronal pulp

Answer (*b*).

Gingival abscess or parulis (gum boil) is because of the degenerated pulp or necrosed pulp.

6. The proximity of carious lesions to the pulp cannot always be determined accurately in the x-ray film. What often appears to be an intact barrier of secondary dentin protecting the pulp may actually be a perforated mass of irregularly calcified and carious material:

(*a*) both the statements are false

(*b*) both the statements are true

(*c*) first statement is true and the second is false

(*d*) first statement is false and the second is true

Answer (*b*).

The answer is self-explanatory.

7. Which of the following conditions are relative contraindications for endodontic therapy in children?

(*a*) Susceptibility to subacute bacterial endocarditis.

(*b*) Nephritis.

(*c*) Leukemia.

(*d*) All of the above.

Answer (d).

In case of children with conditions which render them susceptible to subacute bacterial endocarditis or those with nephritis, leukemia, solid tumours or idiopathic cyclic neutropenia, extraction of the involved tooth after proper premedication with antibiotics should be the treatment of choice rather than pulp therapy.

8. The teeth selected for indirect pulp treatment should fulfil which of the following criteria:

(*a*) no history of spontaneous unprovoked toothache

(*b*) no tenderness to percussion

(*c*) no abnormal mobility

(*d*) no radiographic evidence of radicular disease

(*e*) no evidence of internal or external resorption

(*f*) all of the above

Answer (f).

Spontaneous pain indicates irreversible pulpitis. Tenderness to percussion indicates inflammation of the periapical tissues. Abnormal mobility indicates periodontal breakdown. Hence in the above situations, endodontic treatment becomes necessary. Also radiographic evidence of radicular disease, internal or external resorption indicates the need for more invasive procedures.

9. The size of the exposure, the appearance of the pulp and the amount of bleeding are valuable observations in diagnosing the condition of primary pulp. The most favourable condition for vital pulp therapy is the small pinpoint exposure surrounded by sound dentin:

(*a*) both the statements are false

(*b*) both the statements are true

(*c*) first statement is true and the second is false

(*d*) first statement is false and the second is true

Answer (*b*).

The answer is self-explanatory.

10. Which of the following criteria are fulfilled when vital-pulp therapy is carried out?

(*a*) small exposures that have been accidentally produced by trauma or during cavity preparation

(*b*) absence of pain with the possible exception of discomfort caused by the intake of food

(*c*) lack of bleeding at the exposure site as is often the case in a mechanical exposure or an amount of bleeding that would be considered normal in the absence of hyperemic or an inflamed pulp

(*d*) any of the above

Answer (*d*).

All of the above mentioned situations can be treated by vital-pulp therapy.

11. The material of choice for direct-pulp capping in permanent molars is:

(*a*) calcium hydroxide

(*b*) zinc oxide eugenol

(*c*) glass ionomer cement

(*d*) reinforced zinc oxide eugenol (IRM)

Answer (*a*).

Calcium hydroxide stimulates formation of reparative dentin. Hence this is the material of choice for pulp capping.

12. The material of choice for pulpotomy in primary molars is:

(*a*) calcium hydroxide
(*b*) zinc oxide eugenol
(*c*) formocresol or glutaraldehyde
(*d*) reinforced zinc oxide eugenol (IRM)

Answer (*c*).

Formocresol or glutaraldehyde is the material of choice for pulpotomy. Calcium hydroxide should not be used for pulpotomy as it causes internal resorption in primary teeth.

13. The material of choice for pulpotomy in permanent molars is:

(*a*) calcium hydroxide
(*b*) zinc oxide eugenol
(*c*) formocresol or glutaraldehyde
(*d*) reinforced zinc oxide eugenol (IRM)

Answer (*a*).

The material of choice for pulpotomy in permanent teeth is calcium hydroxide because of its ability to induce secondary dentin formation.

14. Who introduced calcium hydroxide?

(*a*) Herman. (*b*) Jordan.
(*c*) Robert Bunon. (*d*) Wilson and Kent.

Answer (*a*).

Wilson and Kent introduced glass ionomer cement in 1972.

15. The pH of calcium hydroxide is:

(*a*) 12 (*b*) 7

(*c*) 3 (*d*) 10

Answer (*a*).

Because of its alkalinity, it is so caustic that when placed in contact with vital-pulp tissue, the reaction produces a superficial necrosis of the pulp.

16. The immediate reaction of the pulp tissue beneath the calcium hydroxide in direct-pulp capping is:

(*a*) inflammation (*b*) necrosis

(*c*) fatty degeneration (*d*) gangrene formation

Answer (*b*).

Refer to the explanation of Q. No. 15.

17. After the pulp-capping procedure, a calcified bridge is evident radiographically in:

(*a*) 2 weeks (*b*) 4 weeks

(*c*) 12 weeks (*d*) 2 months

Answer (*b*).

One month after the pulp-capping procedure a calcified bridge is evident radiographically. This bridge continues to increase in thickness during the next 12-month period. The pulp tissue beneath the calcified bridge remains vital and is essentially free of inflammatory cells.

18. Which of the following is not an advantage of glutaraldehyde over formocresol as a pulpotomy agent?

(*a*) Formaldehyde reactions are reversible but glutaraldehyde reactions are not.

(*b*) Formaldehyde is a small molecule that penetrates the apical foramen, whereas glutaraldehyde is a larger molecule that does not.

(*c*) Formaldehyde requires a long reaction time and an excess of solution to fix tissue, whereas glutaraldehyde fixes tissue instantly and excess solution is not required.

(*d*) The amount of glutaraldehyde absorbed systemically is more.

Answer (*d*).

The systemic absorption of glutaraldehyde is less when compared to formocresol. Hence the fourth choice is not correct regarding glutaraldehyde.

19. The concentration of glutaraldehyde used for pulpotomy is:

(*a*) 4% (*b*) 8%

(*c*) 2% (*d*) 6%

Answer (*c*).

The answer is self-explanatory.

20. Which of the following is an indication of failure after vital-pulp therapy:

(*a*) internal resorption

(*b*) alveolar abscess

(*c*) early exfoliation after pulp treatment

(*d*) any of the above

Answer (*d*).

Radiographic evidence of internal resorption occurring within the pulp canal several months after pulpotomy procedure is the most frequently seen evidence of an abnormal response in primary teeth. An alveolar abscess occasionally develops some months after the pulp therapy has been completed. The child may present with a fistulous opening indicating the chronicity of the infection. Occasionally a pulpally treated tooth previously believed to be successfully managed will loosen and exfoliate prematurely for no reason. It is believed that such a condition results from low grade, chronic, asymptomatic and localized infection.

Chapter 12

Local Anesthesia and Surgical Considerations

1. The most effective topical anesthetic is:

(*a*) lignocaine

(*b*) tetracaine

(*c*) ethyl amino benzoate

(*d*) dyclonine

Answer (*c*).

Benzocaine is the most effective topical anesthetic. It is otherwise known as ethyl amino benzoate. It has a rapid onset and longer duration of anesthesia than the other topical agents.

2. Jet injection was introduced by:

(*a*) Figge and Scherer (1947)

(*b*) Schroeder (1948)

(*c*) McKay (1952)

(*d*) Frank (1966)

Answer (*a*).

The jet injection is based on the principle that small quantities of liquids forced through very small openings under high pressure can penetrate the mucous membrane or skin without causing excessive trauma.

3. All of the following are true regarding jet injection (Syrijet) except:

(*a*) it is based on the principle that small quantities of liquids forced through very small openings under high pressure can penetrate mucous membrane or skin without causing excessive trauma.

(*b*) it produces surface anesthesia instantly.

(*c*) it can be used for obtaining gingival anesthesia before rubber dam placement.

(*d*) it cannot be employed in the place of needle injection for nasopalatine and long buccal nerve blocks.

Answer (*d*).

Jet injection (Syrijet) can be used in the place of needle injection for nasopalatine and long buccal nerve blocks.

4. Mandibular foramen is situated at a level lower than the occlusal plane of primary teeth of the pediatric patient. Therefore the injection must be made slightly higher and more anteriorly than that for an adult patient.

(*a*) Both the statements are false.

(*b*) Both the statements are true.

(*c*) First statement is true and the second is false.

(*d*) First statement is false and the second is true.

Answer (*c*).

Mandibular foramen is situated at a level lower than the occlusal plane of primary teeth of the pediatric patient. Therefore the injection must be made slightly lower and more posteriorly than for an adult patient.

5. Long buccal nerve block is needed for placement of a rubber dam clamp in molars. To obtain long buccal nerve block small quantity of solution is deposited in the mucobuccal fold at a point distal and buccal to the indicated tooth.

(*a*) Both the statements are false.

(*b*) Both the statements are true

(*c*) First statement is true and the second is false.

(*d*) First statement is false and the second is true.

Answer (*b*).

The answer is self-explanatory.

6. Gow Gates mandibular block technique anesthetizes all except:

(*a*) mandibular molars (*b*) mylohyoid

(*c*) premolars (*d*) mandibular incisors

Answer (*d*).

This single injection anesthetizes the entire right or left half of the mandibular teeth and soft tissues except the incisors which may receive partial innervation from the incisive nerves of the opposite side.

7. In a child with only primary dentition erupted, the injection for greater palatine block should be made approximately 30 mm posterior to the distal surface of the second primary molar. The innervation of soft tissue

of posterior two third of palate is derived from the greater and lesser palatine nerves.

(*a*) Both the statements are false.

(*b*) Both the statements are true.

(*c*) First statement is true and the second is false.

(*d*) First statement is false and the second is true.

Answer (*d*).

The injection for greater palatine block should be given 10 mm posterior to the distal surface of the second primary molar.

8. The preferred block for a surgical removal of impacted canines in a child is:

(*a*) supra periosteal injection

(*b*) posterior and middle superior nerve block

(*c*) infra orbital nerve block

(*d*) mental nerve block

Answer (*c*).

Infra orbital nerve block anesthetizes anterior and middle superior alveolar nerves. It also affects innervation of the soft tissues below the eye, half of the nose and the oral musculature of the upper lip on the injected side of the face.

9. In intraligamentary injection the needle is placed in the gingival sulcus usually on the mesial surface and advanced along the root surface until resistance is met. Then 0.2 ml of solution is deposited into the periodontal ligament:

(*a*) both the statements are false

(*b*) both the statements are true

(*c*) first statement is true and the second is false

(*d*) first statement is false and the second is true

Answer (*b*).

The question explains the technique of intra ligamentary injection. For multirooted teeth, injections are made both mesially and distally. This technique is useful in patients with bleeding disorders that contradict other injections.

10. Which of the following are advantages of intraligament injection technique?

(*a*) Provides reliable pain control rapidly and easily.

(*b*) It provides pulpal anesthesia for 30–45 minutes.

(*c*) It may be useful in patients with bleeding disorders that contraindicate other injection.

(*d*) It may be useful in young or disabled patients in whom the problems of postoperative trauma to the lips or tongue is a concern.

(*e*) All of the above.

Answer (*e*).

The answer is self-explanatory.

11. The British-styled extraction forceps differ from American designed forceps, especially those for the lower teeth. The British system of exodontia usually employs a stand up posture and the force is applied via the whole forearm whereas in the American system it is via wrist action:

(*a*) both the statements are true

(*b*) both the statements are false

(*c*) first statement is true and the second is false

(*d*) first statement is false and the second is true

Answer (*a*).

The answer is self-explanatory.

12. All of the following are amide group of local anesthetic agents except:

(*a*) Lignocaine (*b*) Mepivacaine

(*c*) Bupivacaine (*d*) Procaine

Answer (*d*).

The answer is self-explanatory. Procaine is an ester type of local anesthetic agent.

13. The maximum dose of lignocaine which can be administered is:

(*a*) 4.4 mg/kg body weight

(*b*) 2 mg/kg body weight

(*c*) 6.4 mg/kg body weight

(*d*) 2 gm/kg body weight

Answer (*a*).

The answer is self-explanatory.

14. All of the following local anesthetic agents are vasodilators except:

(*a*) Lignocaine

(*b*) Bupivacaine

(*c*) Mepivacaine

(*d*) Cocaine

Answer (*d*).

Cocaine is the only local anesthetic that consistently produces vasoconstriction. The initial action of cocaine is vasodilation, which is followed by an intense and prolonged vasoconstriction.

15. Which of the following are used in a traditional local anesthetic solution?

(*a*) Vehicle. (*b*) Fungicide.

(*c*) Preservative. (*d*) All of the above.

Answer (*d*).

The fungicide used in local anesthetic solution is thymol and the preservative is methylparaben. The vehicle is usually water.

Chapter 13

Gingival and Periodontal Diseases in Children

1. Which of the following is true about gingiva?

(*a*) Gingiva is that part of oral mucous membrane that covers the alveolar processes and the cervical portions of the teeth.

(*b*) Free gingiva is the tissue coronal to the bottom of the gingival sulcus.

(*c*) Attached gingiva is the tissue which extends apically from where the free gingiva ends up to the mucogingival junction.

(*d*) All of the above.

Answer (*d*).

The three choices given above define gingiva, free gingiva and attached gingiva, respectively.

2. The colour of the gingiva is determined by:

(*a*) complexion of the person

(*b*) thickness of the tissue

(*c*) degree of keratinization

(*d*) all of the above

Answer (*d*).

The gingival tissues are normally light pink in colour. But the colour is usually related to any of the three factors mentioned above. In a healthy adult, the marginal gingiva has a sharp knife like edge; during the period of eruption in the child, however, the gingiva is thicker and has rounded margins.

3. Gingivitis is an inflammation involving only the gingival tissues next to the tooth. Microscopically it is characterized by the presence of inflammatory exudates and edema, some destruction of collagenous gingival fibres and ulceration and proliferation of the epithelium facing the tooth and attaching the gingiva to it.

(*a*) Both the statements are false.

(*b*) Both the statements are true.

(*c*) First statement is true and the second is false.

(*d*) First statement is false and the second is true.

Answer (*b*).

The answer is self-explanatory.

4. All of the following about plaque is true except:

(*a*) it is a complex entity

(*b*) metabolically interconnected, highly disorganized bacterial system

(*c*) it consists of dense masses of microorganisms

(*d*) it also has an intermicrobial matrix

Answer (*b*).

Plaque is considered to be a complex, metabolically interconnected, highly organized bacterial system consisting of dense masses of microorganisms embedded in an intermicrobial matrix.

5. Plaque begins to form on tooth surface after brushing in:

(*a*) 4 hours

(*b*) 6 hours

(*c*) 8 hours

(*d*) 2 hours

Answer (*d*).

Plaque begins to form within 2 hours after the teeth are brushed. Coccus bacteria form on the pellicle first. Within 5 hours, plaque microcolonies develop by cell division. Between 6–12 hours the covering material becomes thinner and is reduced to small-scattered areas. Rod-shaped bacteria appears for the first time in 24 hours old plaque. Within 48 hours, rods and filaments cover the surface of the plaque.

6. Supragingival calculus occurs as soft, firmly adherent masses on the crowns of teeth. Subgingival calculus is found as a concretion on the tooth in the confines of the periodontal pocket.

(*a*) Both the statements are false.

(*b*) Both the statements are true.

(*c*) First statement is true and the second is false.

(*d*) First statement is false and the second is true.

Answer (*d*).

Supragingival calculus occurs as hard, firmly adherent masses on the crowns of the teeth.

7. All of the following are true regarding eruption gingivitis except:

(*a*) it is not seen during the eruption of primary teeth

(*b*) it is usually seen during the eruption of 1st and 2nd permanent molars

(*c*) it can lead to pericoronitis or a pericoronal abscess

(*d*) it occurs because the gingival margin receives no protection from the coronal contour of the tooth during the early stages of active eruption. Also the continual impingement of food on the gingiva causes the inflammatory process

Answer (*a*).

It is often observed in young children when the primary teeth are erupting. This gingivitis often associated with difficult eruption subsides after the teeth emerge into the oral cavity. The greatest increase in the incidence of gingivitis in children is again seen in the 6–7 years group when the permanent teeth begin to erupt.

8. Which of the following is true of acute herpetic gingivostomatiits?

(*a*) It is caused by HSV-1.

(*b*) 99% of all primary infection is of sub-clinical type.

(*c*) It usually affects preschool children.

(*d*) All of the above.

Answer (*d*).

The answer is self-explanatory.

9. The active symptoms of acute herpetic gingivostomatitis are:

(*a*) malaise, irritability, headache

(*b*) pain associated with intake of food and liquids

(*c*) presence of yellow or white liquid filled vesicles

(*d*) all of the above

Answer (*d*).

The active symptoms can occur in children with clean mouth and healthy oral tissues. These children are as susceptible as those with poor oral hygiene. All the above mentioned symptoms develop suddenly.

10. Acute herpetic gingivostomatitis in children runs a course of 10–14 days. Treatment should be directed towards the relief of the acute symptoms so that fluid and nutritional intake can be maintained.

(*a*) Both the statements are false.

(*b*) Both the statements are true.

(*c*) First statement is true and the second is false.

(*d*) First statement is false and the second is true.

Answer (*b*).

The answer is self-explanatory.

11. Which of the following is a treatment for acute herpetic gingivostomatitis?

(*a*) Application of topical anesthetics like dyclonine hydrochloride (0.5%).

(*b*) Application of a mixture of diphenhydramine elixir and kaopectate.

(*c*) Lidocaine topical application.

(*d*) Any of the above.

Answer (*d*).

Application of a mild topical anesthetic like dyclonine hydrochloride before mealtime will temporarily relieve the pain and allow the child to take a soft diet. Diphenhydramine has mild analgesic and anti-inflammatory properties whereas kaopectate coats the lesions.

12. All of the following are true about recurrent herpes labialis (RHL) except:

(*a*) HSV 1 virus remains in the sensory ganglia and reappears later as RHL

(*b*) the sore essentially occurs on the lips

(*c*) emotional stress and lowered tissue resistance are not related to this condition

(*d*) it can appear after dental treatment and may be related to irritation from rubber dam

Answer (*c*).

The recurrent form of disease is often related to conditions of emotional stress and lowered tissue resistance resulting from various types of trauma. Excessive exposure to sunlight, irritation from rubber dam during dental treatment can also precipitate recurrent herpes labialis.

13. Recurrent aphthous ulcer is otherwise called:

(*a*) canker sore

(*b*) cold sore

(*c*) recurrent herpes labialis

(*d*) recurrent herpetic infection

Answer (*a*).

Recurrent aphthous ulcer is otherwise called canker sore or recurrent aphthous stomatitis. Recurrent aphthous stomatitis is characterized by recurrent ulcerations on the moist mucous membranes of the mouth in which both discrete and confluent lesions are found rapidly in certain sites and they feature a round to oval crateriform base, raised reddened margins with pain.

14. In a review of aphthous ulcer, it is suggested that the precipitating factor accountable for as much as 75% of episodes is minor trauma. Nutritional deficiencies are found in 20% people with aphthous ulcer.

(*a*) Both the statements are true.

(*b*) Both the statements are false.

(*c*) The first statement is true and the second is false.

(*d*) The first statement is false and the second is true.

Answer (*a*).

Injuries caused by cheek biting and minor facial irritations are probably the most common precipitating factors. The clinically detectable nutritional deficiencies include iron, Vitamin B_{12} and folic acid. Stress may also prove to be an important precipitating factor particularly in stress-prone group such as students in professional schools and military personnel.

15. Which of the following is true regarding ANUG?

(*a*) It is characterized by involvement of interproximal gingiva and the presence of a pseudomembranous necrotic covering over the marginal tissue.

(*b*) It is caused by Borrelia Vincentii and fusiform bacilli referred to as spirochetal organisms.

(*c*) Fever, malaise, fetid odour, painful bleeding gingival tissues and poor appetite are other features.

(*d*) The disease responds within 24–48 hours to subgingival curettage, debridement and the use of mild oxidizing solutions.

(*e*) All of the above.

Answer (*e*).

All of the above mentioned facts are true regarding ANUG.

16. The enlargement of the gingival tissues in puberty gingivitis is confined to the anterior segment and may be present in only one arch. The lingual gingival tissue generally remains unaffected.

(*a*) Both the statements are true.

(*b*) Both the statements are false.

(*c*) The first statement is true and the second is false.

(*d*) The first statement is false and the second is true

Answer (*a*).

Puberty gingivitis occasionally develops in children in the prepubertal and pubertal period. Treatment of puberty gingivitis should be improved oral hygiene, removal of all local irritants, restoration of carious teeth and dietary recommendations necessary to ensure an adequate nutritional status.

17. In elephantiasis gingivae, the gingival tissues appear normal at birth but begin to enlarge with the eruption of the primary teeth. During surgical removal of the enlarged gingiva excessive hemorrhage is seen.

(*a*) Both the statements are true.

(*b*) Both the statements are false.

(*c*) The first statement is true and the second is false.

(*d*) The first statement is false and the second is true.

Answer (*a*).

Elephantiasis gingivae or hereditary hyperplasia of the gums is a rare type of gingivitis. Though the enlarged gingiva appears pale and firm, the surgical procedure is accompanied by excessive hemorrhage.

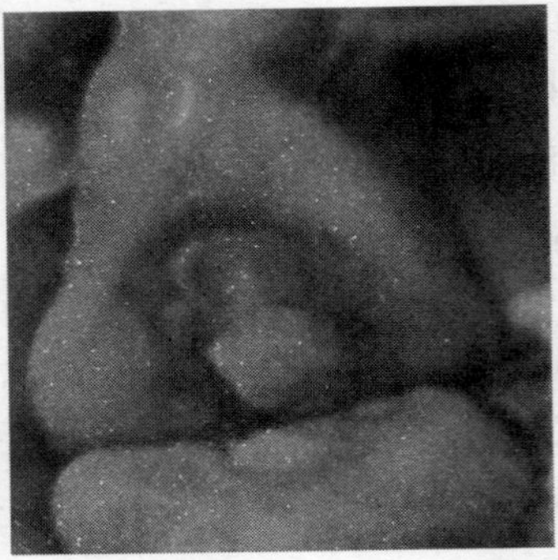

Fig. 13.1 Elephantiasis gingivae.

18. How early is gingival enlargement expected once phenytoin therapy is initiated?

(*a*) 2–3 days

(*b*) 2–3 weeks

(*c*) 2–3 months

(*d*) 24–48 hours

Answer (*b*).

Phenytoin was first introduced as anticonvulsant in 1938 by Merrit and Putnam. Kimball first described gingival hyperplasia as a side effect of this drug in 1939. Phenytoin induced gingival overgrowth (PIGO) or dilantin hyperplasia begins to appear as early as 2–3 weeks after initiation of phenytoin therapy and peaks at 18–24 months.

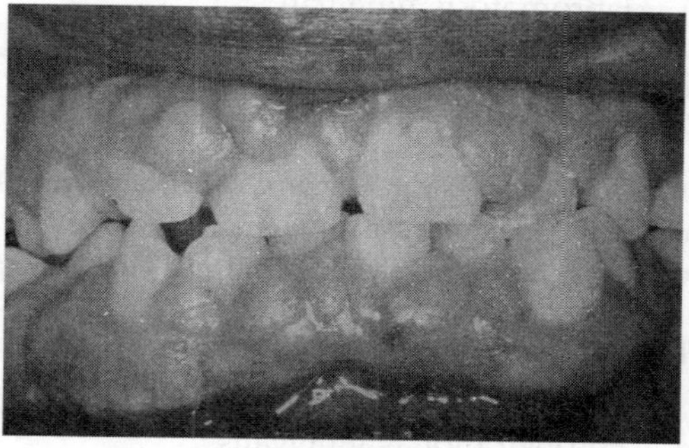

Fig. 13.2 Phenytoin induced gingival overgrowth.

19. The initial clinical appearance of phenytoin induced gingival enlargement is painless enlargement of interproximal gingiva in which buccal and anterior segment are more affected than the lingual and posterior segments. Unless secondary inflammation is present the gingiva appears firm and does not bleed easily upon probing.

(*a*) Both the statements are true.

(*b*) Both the statements are false.

(*c*) The first statement is true and the second is false.

(*d*) The first statement is false and the second is true.

Answer (*a*).

The answer is self-explanatory.

20. Which of the following gingival enlargement is primarily a capillary disease (In which the endothelium swells and degenerates)?

(*a*) Scorbutic gingivitis.

(*b*) Phenytoin induced gingival enlargement.

(*c*) Fibromatosis gingivae.

(*d*) Puberty gingivitis.

Answer (*a*).

Gingivitis associated with vitamin C deficiency is called scorbutic gingivitis. The child usually complains of severe pain and spontaneous hemorrhage will be evident on the gingivae.

21. Which of the following microorganisms is/are involved in juvenile periodontitis?

(*a*) Porphyromonas gingivalis.

(*b*) Bacteroides melaninogenicus.

(*c*) Fusobacterium nucleatum.

(*d*) Actinobacillus actinomycetemcomitans.

(*e*) All of the above.

Answer (*e*).

Localized juvenile periodontitis is associated with Bacteroides melaninogenicus and Actinobacillus actinomycetemcomitans whereas generalized juvenile periodontitis is associated with porphyromonas gingivalis and Actinobacillus actinomycetem-comitans.

22. Frenectomy involves complete excision of the frenum and its periosteal attachment. A frenotomy involves incision of the periosteal fibre attachment and possibly suturing of the frenum to the periosteum at the base of the mandible.

(*a*) Both the statements are true.

(*b*) Both the statements are false.

(*c*) The first statement is true and the second is false.

(*d*) The first statement is false and the second is true.

Answer (*a*).

A frenum is a membranous fold that joins two parts and restricts the individual movements of each. The question defines frenectomy and frenotomy procedures.

23. A mandibular frenum that inhibits the tongue from touching the maxillary central incisor would interfere with the childs ability to make 't', 'd' and 'l' sounds. As long as the child has enough range of motion to raise the tongue to the roof of the mouth no surgery would be indicated.

(*a*) Both the statements are true.

(*b*) Both the statements are false.

(*c*) The first statement is true and the second is false.

(*d*) The first statement is false and the second is true.

Answer (*a*).

Some commonly observed locations of frenums in the child are on the facial gingival surface of the anterior midline of the maxilla, on the facial and lingual gingival surfaces of the anterior midline of the mandible and on the mandibular and maxillary premolar facial area.

24. PMA index assesses:

(*a*) the amount of calculus

(*b*) gingivitis

(*c*) periodontal status

(*d*) the marginal gingiva specifically

Answer (*b*).

The answer is self-explanatory.

25. The teeth usually examined in the simplified oral hygiene index are:

(*a*) molars and premolars

(*b*) molars and incisors

(*c*) premolars and incisors

(*d*) incisors and canines

Answer (*b*).

Molars and incisors are usually examined in simplified oral hygiene index.

26. PMA index was given by:

(*a*) Greene and Vermilion

(*b*) Massler and Schour

(*c*) Moore

(*d*) Russell

Answer (*b*).

Massler and Schour introduced the PMA index (papillary marginal and attached gingival index). Russell introduced the periodontal index.

Different types of stains

S. No.	*Stain*	*Features*
1.	Green stain	Seen in young people. Cause unknown (may be due to chromogenic bacteria). Seen in gingival third of labial surface of maxillary anterior teeth. Commonly seen in labial surface of mouth breathers. Enamel beneath the stain might have undergone initial demineralization.
2.	Orange	Occurs less frequently than green stain. Cause unknown. Often seen in gingival third of the tooth and is associated with poor oral hygiene.
3.	Black	Less common than orange and green stain. Seen as a line following gingival contour or it may be generalized (usually on rough and pitted areas). Children with black stains are usually caries free.

Chapter 14

Traumatic Injuries

1. A dental disturbance that has a greater psychological impact on both the parents and the child is:

(*a*) multiple decayed teeth

(*b*) discolored front tooth

(*c*) fracture or loss of a anterior tooth

(*d*) mucocele

Answer (*c*).

Fracture or loss of an anterior tooth due to trauma is a tragic experience for the young patient as well as the parents.

2. Facial fractures in children has a very low incidence because:

(*a*) of the elastic nature of the child's facial bones

(*b*) lack of exposure to alcohol associated motor-vehicle accidents

(*c*) anatomic protection offered by prominent calveria

(*d*) any of the above

Answer (*d*).

All of the above factors contribute to the decreased incidence of facial fractures in children. Because of the resilient bones surrounding the primary teeth, injuries usually comprise tooth luxations.

3. A fracture can be defined as a sudden violent breach of continuity of bone, which may be complete or incomplete in character. Contusion is produced by blunt trauma that results in edema and hematoma formation in the subcutaneous tissues.

(*a*) Both the statements are true.

(*b*) Both the statements are false.

(*c*) The first statement is true and the second is false.

(*d*) The first statement is false and the second is true.

Answer (*a*).

The question defines fracture and contusion.

4. An abrasion results from friction along a surface, removing or peeling of the superficial layers of the skin that results in a raw exposed or bleeding surface. On the other hand, laceration is one, which causes a discontinuity in the skin or mucosal surface, which can be simple, stellate, jagged, beveled, or flaplike.

(*a*) Both the statements are true.

(*b*) Both the statements are false.

(*c*) The first statement is true and the second is false.

(*d*) The first statement is false and the second is true.

Answer (*a*).

The question differentiates abrasion from laceration.

5. Which of the following is the most common injury in the oro-facial region?

(*a*) Laceration (*b*) Contusion
(*c*) Abrasion (*d*) Avulsion

Answer (*a*).

Laceration is the most common injury after trauma to the oro-facial region.

6. Trauma to primary dentition occurs most commonly in ____________ age group:

(*a*) less than 1 year
(*b*) 1–2.5 years
(*c*) 2.5–3.5 years
(*d*) 4–6 years

Answer (*b*).

Trauma to primary dentition occurs most commonly in 1–2.5 years age group because the child starts walking between 10–20 months during which child falls frequently.

7. Children with accident-prone facial profiles belong to ____________ category of malocclusion:

(*a*) Class I (*b*) Class II div. 1
(*c*) Class II div. 2 (*d*) Class III

Answer (*b*).

Injuries to the teeth are common in children with protruding anterior teeth. In Class II div. 1 malocclusion the protrusion of maxillary incisors makes these teeth more susceptible to injury.

8. Children with cerebral palsy are a special group with more predilections to dental trauma. This is because many children with cerebral palsy have protruding anterior teeth and they are subject to frequent falls.

(*a*) Both the statements are true.

(*b*) Both the statements are false.

(*c*) The first statement is true and the second is false.

(*d*) The first statement is false and the second is true.

Answer (*a*).

The answer is self-explanatory.

9. All of the following are true of direct trauma except:

(*a*) when the tooth itself is struck against a surface or when an object strikes a tooth or teeth

(*b*) example for direct trauma is hitting against a table, a chair or in a playground

(*c*) this usually involves anterior dentition

(*d*) this type of trauma also favours crown or crown-root fractures in the premolar or molar region; also possibility of jaw fractures

Answer (*d*).

Indirect trauma such as injuries to chin transmits the forces to the posterior teeth resulting in crown or crown-root fractures in the premolar or molar region.

10. High-velocity blows cause the greatest damage to the supporting structures of the dentition but tooth fractures are less frequent. Low-velocity impacts result in crown-fractures and are usually not associated with damage to the supporting structures.

(*a*) Both the statements are true.

(*b*) Both the statements are false.

(*c*) The first statement is true and the second is false.

(*d*) The first statement is false and the second is true.

Answer (*b*).

The reverse is true. Low-velocity blows cause the greatest damage to the supporting structures of the dentition but tooth fractures are less frequent. High-velocity impacts result in crown fractures and are usually not associated with damage to the supporting structures.

11. All of the following factors involved in traumatic injury to the teeth are described correctly except:

(*a*) sharp impact favours clean crown fractures with minimum tooth displacement because the energy is spread rapidly over a limited area

(*b*) enamel is fractured easily when the direction of impacting force is parallel to the enamel rods and with dentin. It fractures easily when the force is perpendicular to the dentinal tubules

(*c*) low-velocity impact causes more tooth fractures than damage to the supporting tissues

(*d*) if a tooth is struck with a resilient or cushioned object the risk of luxation and alveolar fracture is increased

Answer (*c*).

Refer to the explanation of Q. No. 10.

12. In the primary dentition, teeth are more frequently displaced or luxated than they are fractured. This is because the alveolar bone in the young child has large marrow spaces and is relatively pliable.

(*a*) Both the statements are true.

(*b*) Both the statements are false.

(*c*) The first statement is true and the second is false.

(*d*) The first statement is false and the second is true.

Answer (*a*).

The alveolar bone in the young child is more elastic and resilient. Hence, it can absorb forces and allow displacement or luxation more frequently.

13. Whose classification of traumatic injuries is based on the system adopted by WHO in its application of International Classification of Diseases to dentistry and stomatology:

(*a*) Rabinowitch 1956

(*b*) Ellis and Davey 1960

(*c*) Andreasen 1981

(*d*) Ulfohn 1985

Answer (*c*).

Andreasen's classification of traumatic injuries is based on WHO classification of injuries to teeth. Classification of traumatic injuries to teeth:

A. Rabinowitch

1. Fractures of enamel/slightly into dentin
2. Fractures into the dentin
3. Fractures into the pulp
4. Fractures of the root
5. Comminuted fractures
6. Displaced teeth

B. Ulfohn

1. Fracture of enamel.
2. Fracture of the crown with indirect-pulp exposure through the dentin.
3. Fracture of the crown with direct-pulp exposure.

C. Ellis and Davey

Class 1 – Simple fracture of the crown involving enamel and little or no dentin.

Class II – Extensive fracture of the crown, involving considerable dentin but not the dental pulp.

Class III – Extensive fracture of the crown, involving considerable dentin and exposing the dental pulp.

Class IV – Traumatised teeth that become nonvital with or without loss of crown structure.

Class V – Teeth lost as a result of trauma.

Class VI – Fracture of the root with or without loss of crown structure.

Class VII – Displacement of a tooth without fracture of crown or root.

Class VIII – Fracture of crown en-masse and its replacement.

Class IX – Traumatic injuries to deciduous teeth.

14. Teeth lost as a result of trauma is classified by Ellis and Davey as:

(*a*) Class I (*b*) Class VII
(*c*) Class VI (*d*) Class V

Answer (*d*).

Refer to the explanation of Q. No. 13.

15. Non-vital teeth belong to ____________ of Ellis and Davey's classification:

(*a*) Class I (*b*) Class VI
(*c*) Class IV (*d*) Class VIII

Answer (*c*).

Refer to the explanation of Q. No. 13.

16. Accident in which a child has fallen with an object in mouth results in:

(*a*) a crown-root fracture

(*b*) dislocation of the teeth in a labial direction

(*c*) fracture of root without crown fracture

(*d*) fracture of crown en-masse

Answer (*b*).

The object in the mouth tends to displace the anterior teeth in a labial direction.

17. Subconjunctival hemorrhage with periorbital ecchymosis and edema suggests a fracture of zygoma, nasal bone or frontal bone. Sublingual hematoma is diagnostic of mandibular fracture.

(*a*) Both the statements are true.

(*b*) Both the statements are false.

(*c*) The first statement is true and the second is false.

(*d*) The first statement is false and the second is true.

Answer (*a*).

The answer is self-explanatory.

18. When deviation of the mandible is seen during opening and closing movements, zygomatic arch fracture should be suspected. Trismus or inability to close the mouth may be an indication of a condylar injury.

(*a*) Both the statements are true.

(*b*) Both the statements are false.

(*c*) The first statement is true and the second is false.

(*d*) The first statement is false and the second is true.

Answer (*b*).

Deviation of the mandible is seen during opening and closing movements in condylar injuries. Trismus or inability to close the mouth may be indicative of a depressed zygomatic arch fracture.

19. Following a trauma, if the tooth reacts to hot, cold, sweet or sour food it indicates exposure of dentin or pulp. If there is sensitivity to pressure on eating or touch it suggests an occlusal disturbance.

(*a*) Both the statements are true.

(*b*) Both the statements are false.

(*c*) The first statement is true and the second is false.

(*d*) The first statement is false and the second is true.

Answer (*a*).

The answer is self-explanatory.

20. Match the following:

	View		*Fracture location*
A.	Water's view	1.	Frontal sinus, frontal bone, ethmoidal cells, zygomatic frontal suture
B.	Caldwell view	2.	Body of the mandible, angle
C.	Towne's view	3.	Condyle, alveolar segment
D.	Panoramic view	4.	Orbital, nasal fracture
E.	Orbital and nasal films	5.	Midface, zygoma, maxilla, maxillary orbital floors and nasal pyramid

(*a*) A-5, B-1, C-2, D-3, E-4

(*b*) A-1, B-2, C-3, D-4, E-5

(*c*) A-3, B-4, C-5, D-2, E-1

(*d*) A-4, B-3, C-5, D-2, E-1

Answer (*a*).

The answer is self-explanatory.

21. Which of the following recent methods are used to assess pulp circulation (vitality)?

(*a*) CT scan

(*b*) MRI

(*c*) Laser doppler flow meter

(*d*) Pulseoximeter

(*e*) (*c*) and (*d*)

Answer (*e*).

Laser doppler flow meter and pulseoximeter are the recent equipments used to assess pulp circulation.

22. The maxilla is the final facial bone to complete normal growth and development. The condylar head is an important growth centre of the mandible.

(*a*) Both the statements are true.

(*b*) Both the statements are false.

(*c*) The first statement is true and the second is false.

(*d*) The first statement is false and the second is true.

Answer (*d*).

The mandible is the final facial bone to complete normal growth and development.

23. Condylar injury before the age of 3 is likely to result in a significant mandibular growth distortion. After 12 years of age, condylar injury has little effect on mandibular growth.

(*a*) Both the statements are true.

(*b*) Both the statements are false.

(*c*) The first statement is true and the second is false.

(*d*) The first statement is false and the second is true.

Answer (*a*).

The answer is self-explanatory.

24. It is not advisable to consider permanent crowning until the child is 17 years. This is because the development of the dentofacial structures would not be complete by then.

(*a*) Both the statements are true.

(*b*) Both the statements are false.

(*c*) The first statement is true and the second is false.

(*d*) The first statement is false and the second is true.

Answer (*a*).

Use of metal ceramic crowns or all ceramic crowns are avoided in children less than 17 years because the final occlusion and gingival margins are not established by that time.

25. In direct-pulp capping, the prime requisite of pulp healing is an adequate seal against oral fluids. Therefore a restoration should be placed immediately, which will protect the pulp-capping material until the healing process is well advanced.

(*a*) Both the statements are true.

(*b*) Both the statements are false.

(*c*) The first statement is true and the second is false.

(*d*) The first statement is false and the second is true.

Answer (*a*).

In other words, after pulp capping a permanent restoration is done in the same visit with cements like GIC, which does not allow marginal leakage. This ensures the success of capping procedure.

26. According to Frank which of the following is a successful result of apexification?

(*a*) Continued closure of the canal and apex to a normal appearance.

(*b*) A dome-shaped apical closure with the canal retaining a blunderbuss appearance.

(*c*) No apparent radiographic change but a positive stop in the apical area.

(*d*) A positive stop and radiographic evidence of a barrier coronal to the anatomic apex of the tooth.

(*e*) Any of the above.

Answer (*e*).

Calcium hydroxide and Mineral trioxide aggregates are some of the materials used to induce apexification. These procedures are carried out in a non-vital tooth. Apexogenesis occurs in a vital tooth where the root end closes physiologically.

27. A tooth receives an injury that causes coronal fracture may have a better pulpal prognosis than a tooth that sustains a severe blow without fracturing the crown. This is because a part of the energy of the blow dissipates as the crown fractures rather than all the energy being absorbed by the tooth's supporting tissues.

(*a*) Both the statements are true.

(*b*) Both the statements are false.

(*c*) The first statement is true and the second is false.

(*d*) The first statement is false and the second is true.

Answer (*a*).

The answer is self-explanatory.

28. A 9-year-old child reports to the office with a maxillary permanent central incisor having a small hypoplastic spot on the labial surface as the chief complaint. The child gives a history of fall when he was 4 years old, which resulted in a fracture of his maxillary primary incisor. The most probable diagnosis is:

(*a*) hypoplasia due to systemic disease

(*b*) fluorosis

(*c*) Turner's tooth

(*d*) amelogenesis imperfecta

Answer (*c*).

Any trauma or infection to primary tooth can result in damage to the succedaneous permanent tooth. This results in hypoplasia of the permanent tooth (Turner's hypoplasia).

29. Primary anterior teeth intruded as the result of a blow may often re-erupt within:

(*a*) 3–4 weeks (*b*) 6–8 weeks

(*c*) 8–12 weeks (*d*) 7–10 days

Answer (*a*).

Treatment of intrusion of a primary teeth is to wait and watch when there is no permanent tooth damage. In such instances the primary tooth re-erupts within 3–4 weeks.

30. Primary teeth that are displaced but not intruded should be repositioned as soon as possible after the accident to prevent interference with occlusion. Frequently the severely loosened primary tooth remains mobile and undergoes rapid root resorption.

(*a*) Both the statements are true.

(*b*) Both the statements are false.

(*c*) The first statement is true and the second is false.

(*d*) The first statement is false and the second is true.

Answer (*a*).

When a primary tooth crown is displaced lingually the apex and cortical bone moves labially (i.e. away from the developing tooth germ). This tooth is left untreated. Over a period of 1–2 months, tongue pressure will reposition the tooth.

31. When a permanent tooth is intruded the tendency for the injury to be followed by rapid root resorption, pulp necrosis or ankylosis is greater. To prevent this from happening, pulp tissue is extirpated and calcium hydroxide is placed inside the root canal as an interim dressing. This is usually done:

(*a*) 2 weeks after the injury

(*b*) 6 weeks after the injury

(*c*) immediately after the trauma (in the first visit itself)

(*d*) 8 weeks after the injury

Answer (*a*).

Intra canal calcium hydroxide has the ability to arrest or delay the onset of external resorption or ankylosis. Hence it is used whenever there is a possibility of ankylosis or external resorption.

32. The success of the replantation procedure is undoubtedly related to the length of time that elapses between the loss of the tooth and its replacement in the socket. The condition of the tooth and particularly the condition of the periodontal ligament tissue remaining on the root surface are also important factors that influence the success of replantation.

(*a*) Both the statements are true.

(*b*) Both the statements are false.

(*c*) The first statement is true and the second is false.

(*d*) The first statement is false and the second is true.

Answer (*a*).

The answer is self-explanatory.

33. Avulsion injuries are more common in children of 7–9 years of age when the incisors are erupting. This is because of the loosely structured periodontal ligament around the erupting teeth which favours complete avulsion.

(*a*) Both the statements are true.

(*b*) Both the statements are false.

(*c*) The first statement is true and the second is false.

(*d*) The first statement is false and the second is true.

Answer (*a*).

The answer is self-explanatory.

34. The best medium to preserve an avulsed tooth is:

(*a*) Milk

(*b*) isotonic saline

(*c*) patients oral cavity

(*d*) HBSS (Hank's balanced salt solution)

Answer (*d*).

The answer is self-explanatory.

35. Primary teeth replantation is contraindicated even in the most ideal conditions. This is because of the poorer prognosis and the additional risk of further injury to the succedaneous tooth.

(*a*) Both the statements are true.

(*b*) Both the statements are false.

(*c*) The first statement is true and the second is false.

(*d*) The first statement is false and the second is true.

Answer (*a*).

In management of traumatic injuries to the primary dentition, the foremost objective is to prevent the damage to the underlying permanent tooth. Any procedure which can cause damage to the permanent tooth, should be avoided.

36. Stabilization by splinting is usually done for 7–14 days after avulsion. Rigid stabilization can induce replacement resorption of the root.

(*a*) Both the statements are true.

(*b*) Both the statements are false.

(*c*) The first statement is true and the second is false.

(*d*) The first statement is false and the second is true.

Answer (*a*).

The different type of injuries and the recommended duration of splinting.

S. No.	*Type of injury*	*Splinting duration*
1.	Subluxation	1–2 weeks
2.	Lateral luxation	4–6 weeks
3.	Root fracture	8–12 weeks

37. All replanted permanent teeth with complete root development should have a pulpectomy soon after replantation regardless of the length of time the tooth was out of the mouth. The pulp is extirpated before the splint is removed preferably within one week after the injury.

(*a*) Both the statements are true.

(*b*) Both the statements are false.

(*c*) The first statement is true and the second is false.

(*d*) The first statement is false and the second is true.

Answer (*a*).

Performance of pulpectomy of an avulsed tooth should be carried out in the mouth within the first week. Pulpectomy should not be carried out in the first visit before replantation as this process prolongs the extra-oral period time of the tooth. Also performing a pulpectomy in a splinted tooth is easier than doing it holding the tooth in hand.

38. In root fractures the best prognosis is with:

(*a*) coronal third fracture

(*b*) middle third fracture

(*c*) apical third fracture

(*d*) fracture between middle and coronal third

Answer (*c*).

Generally apical third fracture of the root does not need any treatment. Middle third fracture may need splinting for 4–6 weeks. Coronal third fracture has the poorest prognosis, as this fracture line tends to communicate with the oral cavity and does not allow healing of it.

39. Following a root fracture, healing takes place by which of the following means:

(*a*) healing with calcified tissue

(*b*) healing with interposition of connective tissue

(*c*) healing with interposition of bone and connective tissue

(*d*) healing with interposition of granulation tissue

(*e*) any of the above

Answer (*e*).

Healing of root fracture can take place by any of the above mentioned means.

40. Which of the following is the least favourable form of repair after root fracture?

(*a*) Healing with calcified tissue.

(*b*) Healing with interposition of connective tissue.

(*c*) Healing with interposition of bone and connective tissue.

(*d*) Healing with interposition of granulation tissue.

Answer (*d*).

Healing with granulation tissue is the least favorable form of healing of a root fracture.

41. A relatively long stabilization period is required for teeth with fractured roots. This seems to encourage the more favourable type of healing with calcified tissue.

(*a*) Both the statements are true.

(*b*) Both the statements are false.

(*c*) The first statement is true and the second is false.

(*d*) The first statement is false and the second is true.

Answer (*a*).

The answer is self-explanatory. Refer to the explanation of Q. No. 40.

42. Splints for root fractures should be more rigid than the splints used for stabilization after other types of displacement injuries. The usual duration for splinting of root fractures is for:

(*a*) 3 months (*b*) 3 weeks

(*c*) 2–3 weeks (*d*) 1 month

Answer (*a*).

Refer to the explanation of Q. No. 36.

43. Which type of tissue necrosis is predominant in oral electrical burns?

(*a*) Fat necrosis.

(*b*) Liquefaction necrosis.

(*c*) Coagulation necrosis.

(*d*) Caseation necrosis.

Answer (*c*).

A common cause of oral burns is electrical trauma. The most frequently encountered electrical injury to children is a burn around the mouth. These burns occur often in children between 6 months and 3 years of age and are equally common among boys and girls.

44. Eschar is:

(*a*) the necrotic tissue after an electrical burn

(*b*) scar tissue which forms after minor oral surgeries like frenectomies

(*c*) scar tissue in the palate

(*d*) an organized clot

Answer (*a*).

Within a few hours after the burn injury there may be a great increase in edema. In 7–10 days the edema begins to subside. The necrotic tissue known as eschar, becomes charred or crusty in appearance and begins to separate from the surrounding viable tissue.

45. After electrical burns, a burn appliance is given to prevent contracture of healing tissue and to serve as a framework on which a normal appearing commissure may be created and preserved. This is usually delivered between:

(*a*) 2–3 days after the injury

(*b*) 10–14 days after injury

(*c*) 6–8 weeks after injury

(*d*) 1–2 days after injury

Answer (*b*).

This burn appliance is given 10–14 days after injury to prevent a contracture and preserve a normal appearing commissure.

46. Which of the following is true about the burn appliance?

(*a*) It has to be worn 24 hours a day for 9–12 months except for eating and cleaning.

(*b*) The appliance is a static base with wings extending laterally to provide contact with both commissures.

(*c*) The shape and location of the wings are important not only in preventing contracture or cohesion of the lips during healing but also in shaping the affected commissure to duplicate the unaffected side.

(*d*) All of the above.

Answer (*d*).

The answer is self-explanatory.

47. Which of the following mouth guards provide a better fit and comfort and are less likely to affect speech?

(*a*) Custom-made mouth guards.

(*b*) Ready-made mouth guards (manufactured and available in the stores).

(*c*) Intraorally-formed mouth guards.

(*d*) All of the above.

Answer (*a*).

Custom-made mouth guards are made from the patient's impression. Hence they provide a better fit and comfort and do not affect speech.

Chapter 15

Eruption of the Teeth

1. The interval between crown completion and the beginning of eruption until the tooth is in full occlusion (for permanent teeth) is approximately:

(*a*) 2 years (*b*) 12 months

(*c*) 3 years (*d*) 5 years

Answer (*d*).

Once the crown formation is completed, the tooth moves through the bone at the rate of 1 mm every 4–6 months. To reach the antagonistic tooth and stabilize itself in occlusion, it takes approximately five years.

2. Extraction of primary molars at 4 or 5 years of age delays the eruption of premolars. Extraction of primary molars at 9 or 10 years of age also delays the eruption of premolars:

(*a*) both the statements are false

(*b*) both the statements are true

(*c*) first statement is true and the second is false

(*d*) first statement is false and the second is true

Answer (*c*).

According to Posen, extraction of primary molars at 4 or 5 years of age delays the eruption of the premolars whereas extraction at 9 or 10 years of age accelerates the eruption of the premolars.

3. Eruption of mandibular second permanent molar before second premolar can cause arch length deficiency. It is desirable that the mandibular canine erupt before the first and second premolars:

(*a*) both the statements are false

(*b*) both the statements are true

(*c*) first statement is true and the second is false

(*d*) first statement is false and the second is true

Answer (*b*).

Eruption of mandibular second permanent molar before second premolar will push the first permanent molar mesially and cause arch length deficiency. In the mandibular arch if the premolar erupts ahead of the canines it can lead to labial positioning of the canines.

4. Which of the following regarding teething is/are true?

(*a*) It is associated with increased salivation.

(*b*) The child puts the hand and fingers into the mouth.

(*c*) Diarrhoea and fever were incorrectly attributed to teething.

(*d*) All of the above.

Answer (*d*).

As teething is a physiological process, its association with fever and systemic disturbances is not justified. Fever or respiratory tract infection at this time should be considered coincidental with the eruption process rather than relating to it. Observations like increased salivation and the child putting the hand and fingers into the mouth may be the only indications that the teeth will soon erupt.

5. Eruption hematoma or eruption cyst is most frequently seen in:

(*a*) primary incisor region

(*b*) primary first molar region

(*c*) primary second molar region

(*d*) primary canine region

Answer (*c*).

Eruption hematoma or cyst-A bluish purple elevated area of tissue develops a few weeks before the eruption of a primary or permanent tooth. This blood filled cyst is most frequently seen in the second primary molar or first permanent molar regions.

6. Eruption sequestrum is usually seen in children during the eruption of:

(*a*) first permanent molar

(*b*) second permanent molar

(*c*) first primary molar

(*d*) second primary molar

Answer (*a*).

A tiny spicule of non viable bone overlying the crown of an erupting permanent molar just before or immediately after the emergence of the tips of the cusps through the oral mucosa is known as the eruption sequestrum.

7. Natal teeth are:

(*a*) teeth that erupt during the first 30 days after birth

(*b*) teeth present at birth
(*c*) teeth that erupt during the first 6 months
(*d*) teeth that erupt 30 days after birth

Answer (*b*).

Natal teeth are teeth which are present at birth and neonatal teeth are the ones which erupt into the oral cavity within the first 30 days after birth.

8. Riga-Fede's disease is characterized by:

(*a*) natal teeth with tongue ulcerations
(*b*) natal teeth with eruption hematoma
(*c*) natal teeth and eruption cyst
(*d*) natal teeth and Epstein pearls

Answer (*a*).

The sharp incisal edges of erupted natal or neonatal teeth may cause laceration of the lingual surface of the tongue. This clinical entity is called Riga-Fede's disease.

9. Most often the natal teeth are:

(*a*) supernumerary primary incisors
(*b*) prematurely erupted primary teeth
(*c*) nothing but dental lamina cyst of newborn
(*d*) none of the above

Answer (*b*).

Zhu and King have reported that 85% of the natal or neonatal teeth are prematurely erupted mandibular primary incisors and only small percentages are supernumerary teeth.

10. Which of the following is/are true regarding ankylosis of primary molars?

(*a*) It follows a familial pattern.

(*b*) It occurs because of missing permanent successors.

(*c*) It occurs because of solid union developing between the bone and the primary teeth during reparative process of resorption.

(*d*) Any of the above.

Answer (*d*).

The answer is self-explanatory.

11. All of the following are true regarding ankylosed teeth except:

(*a*) ankylosis usually occurs in the primary molar region

(*b*) ankylosed teeth are otherwise called submerged teeth

(*c*) if ankylosis occurs early, the involved tooth may lie below the plane of occlusion

(*d*) ankylosis always occurs after the eruption of tooth into the oral cavity

Answer (*d*).

Ankylosis can occasionally occur even before the eruption and complete root formation of primary tooth.

12. Diagnosis of ankylosed tooth can made by the:

(*a*) presence of tooth out of occlusion

(*b*) break in continuity of the periodontal ligament in a radiograph

(*c*) metallic sound while percussing the suspected tooth

(*d*) any of the above

Answer (*d*).

Because eruption has not occurred and the alveolar process has not developed in normal occlusion, the opposing molars in the area seem to be out of occlusion. The ankylosed tooth will have a metallic sound on percussion whereas the normal tooth will have a cushioned-sound because it has an intact periodontal membrane that absorbs some of the shock of the blow. A break in the continuity of the periodontal membrane on a radiograph indicates ankylosis.

13. Which of the following is/are true about Down syndrome?

(*a*) First primary teeth may not appear until 2 years of age.

(*b*) Primary dentition may not be complete until 4–5 years of age.

(*c*) The eruption of teeth often follows an abnormal sequence and some primary teeth may be retained until 14–15 years of age.

(*d*) All of the above.

Answer (*d*).

The answer is self-explanatory.

14. Down syndrome is:

(*a*) trisomy 13 (*b*) trisomy 18

(*c*) trisomy 21 (*d*) trisomy 15

Answer (*c*).

Refer to the table given on next page.

S. No.	Trisomy	Name of the syndrome
1.	13	Patau syndrome
2.	18	Edward syndrome
3.	21	Down syndrome

15. Marie-Sainton syndrome is:

(*a*) achondroplasia

(*b*) ectodermal dysplasia

(*c*) cleidocranial dysplasia

(*d*) hypopituiatarism

Answer (*c*).

Marie-Sainton syndrome is otherwise called cleidocranial dysplasia or osteodentin dysplasia or mutational dysostosis.

16. All of the following are true regarding cleidocranial dysostosis except:

(*a*) absence of clavicles or remnants of clavicles as evidenced by presence of sternal and acromial ends

(*b*) large fontanelles

(*c*) large frontal sinus

(*d*) complete primary dentition at 15 years of age resulting from delayed resorption of the deciduous teeth followed by delayed eruption of permanent teeth is not uncommon

Answer (*c*).

The diagnosis of cleidocranial dysplasia is by the absence of clavicles, as evidenced by the presence of the sternal and acromial ends. The fontanelles are usually large and radiographs of the head show open sutures even late in the child's life. The sinuses particularly the frontal sinus is usually small. Sometimes all the primary teeth are retained till 15 years of age.

17. Multiple supernumerary teeth is characteristic of:

(*a*) cleidocranial dysostosis

(*b*) ectodermal dysplasia

(*c*) dwarfism

(*d*) hyperthyroidism

Answer (*a*).

Some children have few supernumerary teeth in the anterior region of the mouth. Others may have a large number of extra teeth throughout the mouth.

18. Which of the following conditions are usually diagnosed at birth?

(*a*) Hypothyroidism.

(*b*) Hypopituitarism.

(*c*) Achondroplastic dwarfism.

(*d*) All of the above.

Answer (*d*).

Congenital hypothyroidism is the result of an absence or underdevelopment of the thyroid glands and insufficient levels of thyroid hormone. It is routinely diagnosed and corrected at birth because of mandatory blood screening of newborn infants. Hypopituitarism is also diagnosed at birth because of mandatory blood screening of newborn infants. Achondroplastic dwarfism is also diagnosed at birth based on the growth of the extremities.

19. The sequence of eruption of primary teeth is:

(*a*) ABCDE (*b*) ABDCE

(*c*) ACBDE (*d*) ADBCE

Answer (*b*).

The answer is self-explanatory.

20. At birth, gum pads are long enough:

(*a*) to accommodate only primary anteriors

(*b*) to accommodate primary and permanent teeth

(*c*) to accommodate all primary teeth

(*d*) to accommodate primary teeth and first permanent molars

Answer (*c*).

The answer is self-explanatory.

Chapter 16

Cephalometrics

1. Cephalometer was introduced by:

(*a*) Simon

(*b*) Racini and Carerra

(*c*) Broadbent

(*d*) Tweed

Answer (*c*).

Broadbent introduced the cephalometer in 1931. In 1922, Simon introduced gnathostatics, a photographic technique that related the teeth and their respective bony bases to each other as well as to specific craniofacial structures. Racini and Carerra obtained the first X-ray films of the skull by the standard lateral view in 1926. Tweed, Steiner, Ricketts developed the clinical application of cephalometrics and the techniques that permit the observation of discrepancies present in the mandible, maxilla, dental units and soft-tissue profile.

2. While taking a cephalometric radiograph the distance between the subject (mid sagittal plane) and the X-ray tube is:

(*a*) 60 inches

(*b*) 120 inches

(*c*) 180 inches

(*d*) 30 inches

Answer (*a*).

While taking a cephalometric radiograph the head of the subject is stabilized by a cephalostat (head holder) and the X-ray tube is positioned at a distance of 60 inches from the midsagittal plane of the subject.

3. Frankfort horizontal plane is:

(*a*) imaginary line from lower border of nose to lower border of ear

(*b*) imaginary plane from lower border of the orbit to tragus of ear

(*c*) imaginary plane from lower border on nose to tragus of ear

(*d*) imaginary line from upper border of orbit to tragus of ear

Answer (*b*).

Refer the following table describing the cephalometric points and planes.

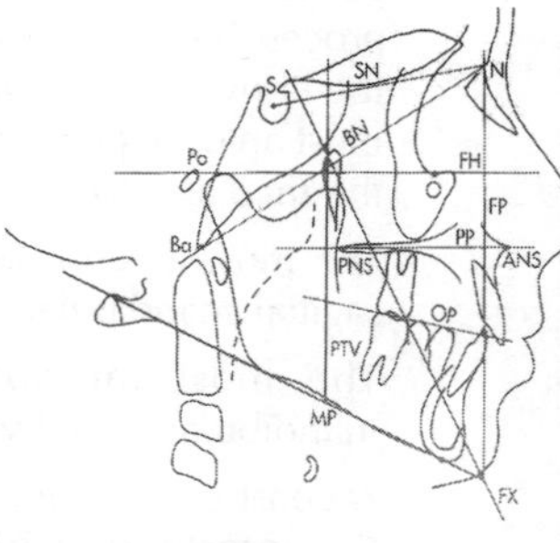

Fig. 16.1 Cephalometric points and planes.

Cephalometric points	*Description*
Sella turcica (S or Sella)	The midpoint of hypophyseal fossa.
Nasion (N)	The external junction of nasofrontal suture in the median plane. If the suture is not visible, this point is located at the deepest concavity of the two bones.
Orbitale (O)	The most inferior point on the external border of the orbit.
Condylion (Cd)	The most superior point on the articular head of the condyle.
Anterior nasal spine (ANS)	The most anterior projection of the anterior nasal spine of the maxilla in the median plane.
A point (subspinale or A)	The deepest point of the curvature of the anterior maxilla between ANS and the alveolar crest. Although A point may change with treatment, it represents the most forward point of the maxilla.
B point (supra-mentale or B)	The most posterior point on the outer curve of the mandibular alveolar process between the alveolar crest and the bony chin. B point delineates the most anterior point of the mandible in the median plane.
Pogonion (Pg)	The most anterior point on the mid-sagittal mandibular symphysis.
Menton (M)	The most inferior point of the mandibular symphysis.
Gnathion (Gn)	A constructed point that is formed by the intersection of the facial and mandibular planes.

Gonion (Go)	A constructed point that is represented by the intersection of the lines tangent to the posterior margin of the ascending ramus and the mandibular plane.
Articulare (Ar)	The point of intersection of the posterior margin of the ascending ramus and the outer margin of the cranial base.
Porion (Po)	A point located at the most superior point of the external auditory meatus or the superior aspect of metal ring that is a component of the left ear rod of the cephalostat.
Basion (Ba)	The most inferior posterior point on the occipital bone that corresponds to the anterior margin of the foramen magnum.
Pterygomaxillary fissure (Ptm)	A teardrop shaped fissure of which the anterior borders of the pterygoid plates of the sphenoid bone create the posterior wall and the anterior wall represents the posterior border of the maxilla (maxillary tuberosity). The tip of the fissure denotes the posterior extent of the maxilla.
Posterior nasal spine (PNS)	The tip of the posterior spine of palatine bone. This landmark is usually not visible on well-exposed lateral head films; therefore it is a constructed point that is represented by the intersection of a continuation of the anterior wall of the pterygopalatine fossa and the floor of the nose. It also denotes the posterior limit of the maxilla.

Pt point (Pt)	The intersection of the inferior border of the foramen rotundum with the posterior wall of Ptm.
CF Point (center of face)	The cephalometric landmark formed by the intersection of the Frankfort horizontal plane and a perpendicular line through Pt.

Cephalometric planes	***Description***
Frankfort horizontal palne (FH)	This plane is constructed from porion to orbitale and represents the basic horizontal plane of the head.
Pterygoid vertical plane (PTV)	A line perpendicular to the Frankfort horizontal plane through the Pt point represents this plane. Studies have shown that the intersection of FH and PTV is very stable, since growth has little effect on this point.
Basion Nasion plane (BN)	This plane passes through basion and nasion. This plane represents cranial base and is the dividing plane between the cranium and the face.
Sella Nasion plane (SN)	A line connecting the sella and the nasion represents this plane. It denotes the antero posterior extent of the anterior cranial base. This reference plane is of questionable diagnostic value in true mandibular prognathism.
Occlusal plane (OP)	This plane separates the mandibular and maxillary permanent molars (or in younger patients the primary second molars) and passes through the contact between the most anterior maxillary and mandibular incisors. If the incisors

	do not contact, the line passes midway between the incisal edges. OP is nearly parallel to both the palatal plane and the Frankfort horizontal plane.
Facial plane (FP)	A line constructed through the nasion perpendicular to the Frankfort horizontal plane represents this plane.
Mandibular plane (MP)	The mandibular plane is constructed as a tangent to the inferior border of the mandible.
Facial axis (FX)	This line is constructed from Pt point through gnathion .FX ideally crosses the basion nasion plane at a right angle.
Palatal plane (PP)	This plane extends through the anterior nasal spine and posterior nasal spine. The relationship of this plane to FH is useful in evaluating treatment changes occurring in the maxilla.

4. The normal SNA is:

(*a*) 90–92 degrees

(*b*) 80–82 degrees

(*c*) 60–62 degrees

(*d*) 70–72 degrees

Answer (*b*).

SNA is the angle between SN plane and A point. The clinical norm for SNA is 82 degrees. This establishes the horizontal location of the maxilla.

5. The normal ANB is:

(*a*) 8–10 degrees

(*b*) 2–4 degrees

(*c*) 12 degrees

(*d*) 0 degrees

Answer (*b*).

ANB is the difference between SNA and SNB angles. The clinical norm for ANB is 2 degrees. This indicates the horizontal relationship between maxilla and mandible. Positive values indicate that the maxilla is forward of the mandible, whereas negative values indicate a Class III skeletal relationship.

6. The normal incisal mandibular plane angle (IMPA) is:

(*a*) 60–64 degrees

(*b*) 90–94 degrees

(*c*) 120–124 degrees

(*d*) 34 degrees

Answer (*b*).

The inner angle between the long axis of the mandibular incisor and mandibular plane. The clinical norm is 90 degrees. This is an evaluation of the angular position of the incisor to the mandibular basal bone.

7. The normal mandibular plane angle (FMA) is:

(*a*) 26 degrees (1 degree decreases every 4 years during normal growth)

(*b*) 26 degrees (1 degree increases every 4 years during normal growth)

(*c*) 46 degrees (4 degree decrease every 2 years during normal growth)

(*d*) 56 degrees (4 degree decrease every 2 years during normal growth)

Answer (*a*).

FMA is the angle formed by the intersection of Frankfurt horizontal plane and mandibular plane. The clinical norm is 26 degrees. This will decrease 1 degree every four years during normal growth. Values in excess of 31 degrees may indicate clockwise growth with dolichofacial growth trends, whereas values less than 21 degrees imply vertical deficiency often seen in brachyfacial growth patterns.

8. Convex facial profile is characteristic of which malocclusion:

(*a*) Class I malocclusion

(*b*) Class II malocclusion (div. 1)

(*c*) Class III malocclusion

(*d*) Class I with crowding

Answer (*b*).

Class I malocclusion generally has a straight profile. Concave profile is characteristic of Class III malocclusion. Convex profile is usually seen in Class II div. 1 malocclusion.

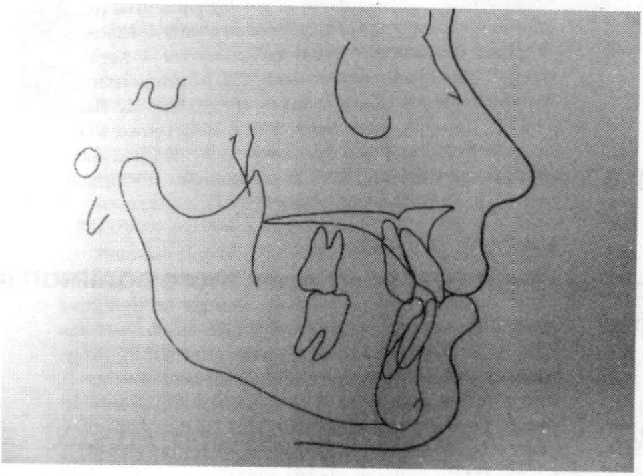

Fig. 16.2 Straight profile.

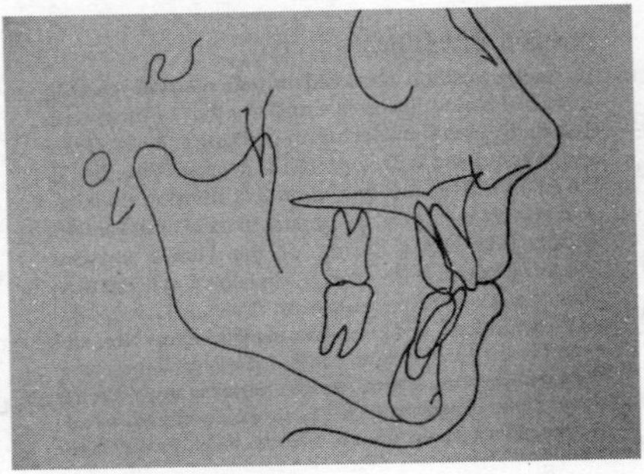

Fig. 16.3 Convex profile.

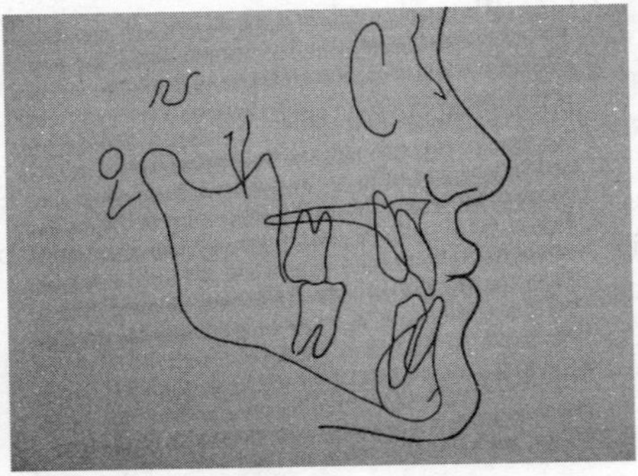

Fig. 16.4 Concave profile.

9. Dolichofacial facial pattern is more common in patients with:

(*a*) Class I malocclusion

(*b*) Class II malocclusion (div. 1)

(*c*) Class III malocclusion

(*d*) Class I with crowding

Answer (*b*).

The faces of these patients are usually long and of weak musculature because of the tendency for vertical growth. The molar occlusion is often of the Class II div. 1 variety.

10. Brachyfacial pattern of face is more common in patients with:

(*a*) Class I malocclusion

(*b*) Class II malocclusion (div. 1)

(*c*) Class III malocclusion

(*d*) Class II malocclusion (div. 2)

Answer (*d*).

The short faces and wide square mandibles of these patients are most often associated with Class II div. II malocclusions. These patients typically exhibit excessive anterior overbites and strong chins.

11. Open bites can be caused by:

(*a*) abnormal habits

(*b*) deviant growth patterns

(*c*) forward tongue position

(*d*) any of the above

Answer (*d*).

Abnormal habits like thumb sucking, digit sucking, tongue thrusting can result in anterior open bite. Forward tongue position can cause anterior open bite, which is more commonly seen in children with Down syndrome.

Chapter 17

Growth and Development

1. Which of the following is not a parameter used in growth literature to assess craniofacial increase?

(*a*) Magnitude

(*b*) Velocity

(*c*) Direction

(*d*) Increment

Answer (*d*).

The parameters commonly used in growth literature to assess the craniofacial size increase are magnitude, velocity and direction. Magnitude refers to the linear dimension overall or that of a part. Direction means the vector of size increase as might be described on a three-dimensional coordinate system. Velocity is defined as the amount of change per unit of time.

2. Which of the following is not characteristic of incremental human growth curve?

(*a*) Rapid accelerating prenatal growth.

(*b*) Rapid accelerating postnatal growth for the first 2–3 years.

(*c*) Period of slow incremental growth during childhood.

(*d*) Growth acceleration for 2–3 years during pubertal adoloscence.

Answer (*b*).

Characteristic of an incremental human growth curve is rapid accelerating prenatal growth, rapid decelerating postnatal growth for the first 2 to 3 years and a period of relatively slow incremental growth during childhood followed by growth acceleration for two or three years during pubertal adolescence.

3. Growth refers to passing from one form (size or shape) to another. Development refers to transitions in functional stage or activity.

(*a*) Both the statements are false.

(*b*) Both the statements are true.

(*c*) First statement is true and the second is false.

(*d*) First statement is false and the second is true.

Answer (*b*).

Growth implies change, a transition from one condition to another. Conceptual growth refers to a passing from one anatomic form (i.e. size and shape) to another. Transitions in functional stage or activity refer to development. Development also means increased organization or specialization of functioning (physiologic) parts.

4. Development refers to:

(*a*) increased specialization or a higher order of organization

(*b*) transition in functional stage or activity

(*c*) progression towards maturity

(*d*) any of the above

Answer (*d*).

The answer is self-explanatory. Refer to the explanation of Q. No. 3.

5. Prenatal period in humans is:

(*a*) 25 weeks in length

(*b*) 40 weeks in length

(*c*) 50 weeks in length

(*d*) 35 weeks in length

Answer (*b*).

S. No.	*Period of growth*	*Duration of the period*
1.	Prenatal period	40 weeks
2.	Infancy	First 2 years after birth
3.	Childhood	2–10 years (Girls) 2–12 years (Boys)
4.	Adolescence	10–18 years (Females) 12–20 years (Males)

6. The period of infancy usually refers to:

(*a*) first 2 years after birth

(*b*) 2–4 years after birth

(*c*) 3–5 years after birth

(*d*) first six months after birth

Answer (*a*).

Refer to the explanation of Q. No. 5.

7. The period of adolescence in humans is:

(*a*) 10–20 years

(*b*) 5–10 years

(*c*) 10–14 years

(*d*) 15–20 years

Answer (*a*).

Refer to the explanation of Q. No. 5.

8. At birth:

(*a*) neural tissue would have attained 30% of adult stature

(*b*) neural tissue would have attained 60–70% of adult stature

(*c*) neural tissue would have attained 90% of adult stature

(*d*) neural tissue would have attained 15% of adult stature

Answer (*b*).

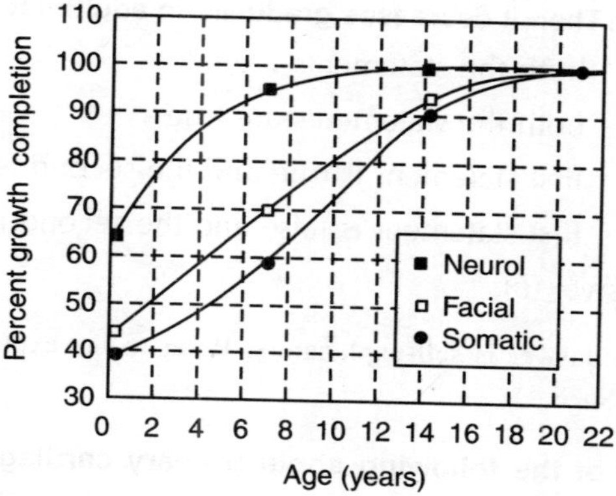

Fig. 17.1 Growth and development of different tissues.

Neural tissue completes its growth at an early stage whereas the general somatic tissues such as muscle, bone and connective tissue mature at a slower rate.

S. No.	Type of tissue	Percentage of growth attained	
		By birth	By middle childhood
1.	Neural tissue	60–70	95
2.	Muscle tissue	40–45	70
3.	Craniofacial lymphoid tissue		125
4.	Craniofacial bone growth	45	70
5.	Craniofacial primary cartilage	75	95

9. The size of craniofacial lymphoid tissue (tonsils and adenoids) is about 125% of adult stature at 5 years of age. Then it decreases gradually to adulthood:

(*a*) both the statements are false

(*b*) both the statements are true

(*c*) first statement is true and the second is false

(*d*) first statement is false and the second is true

Answer (*b*).

The answer is self-explanatory. Refer to the explanation of Q. No. 8.

10. All of the following about primary cartilage is true except:

(*a*) has the capacity for appositional growth

(*b*) pressure tolerant

(*c*) non-vascular

(*d*) does not require a covering membrane for survival

(*e*) is under high genetic control

Answer (*a*).

According to Enlow, cartilage is singular in form, has the capacity to grow from within (interstitial growth), is pressure-tolerant, non calcified, flexible and non-vascular and does not require a covering nutrient membrane for survival. According to Scott, primary cartilage is genetically predisposed, acts during growth as autonomous tissue and is able to directly influence the craniofacial pattern. Appositional growth is characteristic of membranous bones and not of primary cartilage.

11. The adolescent growth spurt is characterized by increased growth velocity at about 10–12 years for females and 12–14 years for males. The maximum velocity or peak-height velocity (PHV) of growth is attained approximately 2 years after pubertal onset.

(*a*) Both the statements are false.

(*b*) Both the statements are true.

(*c*) First statement is true and the second is false.

(*d*) First statement is false and the second is true.

Answer (*b*).

The answer is self-explanatory.

12. During infancy and early childhood the maxilla will be most likely thrusted:

(*a*) backward and downward

(*b*) forward and downward

(*c*) forward and upward

(*d*) backward and upward

Answer (*b*).

The answer is self-explanatory.

13. A mesial step is defined as lower second primary molar mesial to the maxillary second primary molar. Distal step terminal plane is descriptive of a mandibular second primary molar distal to upper second primary molar.

(*a*) Both the statements are false.

(*b*) Both the statements are true.

(*c*) First statement is true and the second is false.

(*d*) First statement is false and the second is true.

Answer (*b*).

The answer is self-explanatory. The incidence of flush terminal plane is 37%, the incidence of mesial step and the distal step being 49% and 14% respectively (See Fig. 17.2).

14. The incidence of end on relationship of the erupting first permanent molars during initial contact is:

(*a*) 27%

(*b*) 49%

(*c*) 23%

(*d*) 1%

Answer (*b*).

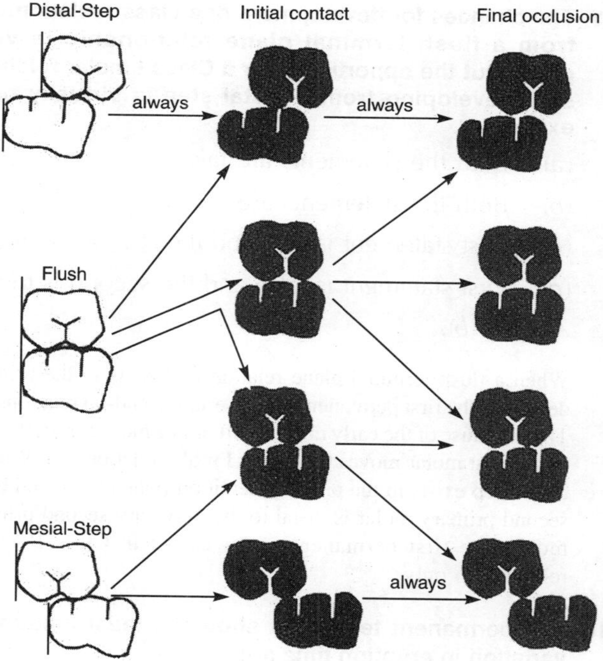

Fig. 17.2 Terminal plane relationship.

S. No.	*Flush terminal plane at age 5 years occlusion*	*Initial first permanent molar*	*Final occlusion at about age 12 years*
1.		1% Class III	3% Class III
2.	49% mesial step	27% Class I	59% Class I
3.	37% flush	49% End-on	
4.	14% distal step	23% Class II	39% Class II

15. The chances for development of a class I relationship from a flush terminal plane relationship is very good. But the opportunity for a Class I molar relationship developing from a distal step is virtually non-existent.

(*a*) Both the statements are false.

(*b*) Both the statements are true.

(*c*) First statement is true and the second is false.

(*d*) First statement is false and the second is true.

Answer (*b*).

When a flush terminal plane relationship exists in the primary dentition, the first permanent molars erupt in end-on relationship. Then because of the early mesial shift or late mesial shift, the first permanent molar moves to a Class I molar relationship. When a distal step exists in the primary dentition (when the mandibular second primary molar is distal to the maxillary second primary molar) the first permanent molar erupts in Class II molar relationship only.

16. The permanent teeth that show the least amount of variation in eruption time are:

(*a*) lower incisors

(*b*) lower second premolars

(*c*) upper first premolars

(*d*) maxillary canines

Answer (*a*).

Eruption time for permanent teeth can vary considerably depending on the specific tooth. According to Garn, eruption time for the lower incisors varies the least; 90% of the lower permanent incisors will erupt within a span of three years. In contrast, with a span of 6.5 years, eruption time varies the most for the lower second premolars.

17. The permanent teeth that show the greatest variation in eruption time:

(*a*) lower incisors

(*b*) lower second premolars

(*c*) upper first premolar

(*d*) maxillary canines

Answer (*b*).

Refer to the explanation of Q. No. 16.

18. If there is a space deficiency of more than 6 mm the treatment of choice is:

(*a*) do nothing; watch

(*b*) lower lingual holding arch

(*c*) space regainers

(*d*) space regainers,arch expansion or extraction

Answer (*d*).

S. No.	*Overall appraisal*	*Space deficiency/ excess in mm*	*Clinical management*
1.	Large space excess	Greater than +3	Long-term planning
2.	Space excess	Less than +3 to 0	Do nothing; watch
3.	Equivalency	0	Watch carefully
4.	Deficiency	Less than 0 to –2	Lower lingual holding arch
5.	Moderate deficiency	–3 to –6	Space regaining or arch expansion
6.	Large deficiency	Greater than –6	Space regaining, arch expansion or extraction

19. Petrovich's hypothesis of craniofacial growth is:

(*a*) Genetic theory

(*b*) Nasal septum theory

(*c*) Functional matrix theory

(*d*) Servo system theory

Answer (*d*).

The theory postulates the influence of somatotrophic hormone–somatomedin complex on the primary and secondary cartilages.

20. An early prepubertal growth spurt indicates:

(*a*) a longer treatment time

(*b*) fast maturing child

(*c*) slow maturing child

(*d*) an endocrine dysfunction

Answer (*b*).

Early prepubertal growth spurt indicates a fast maturing child. In such situations growth modification treatment should be started earlier than normal individuals.

21. The downward and forward direction of facial growth results from:

(*a*) upward and backward growth of the maxillary sutures and the mandibular condyle

(*b*) downward and forward growth of the maxillary sutures and the mandibular condyle

(*c*) interstitial growth in maxilla and mandible

(*d*) vertical eruption and mesial drift of dentitions

Answer (*b*).

The answer is self-explanatory.

22. Which of the following is correct in relation to timing of growth spurt?

(*a*) Boys have earlier growth spurt than girls.

(*b*) Girls have earlier growth spurt than boys.

(*c*) Boys and girls have growth spurts almost at the same time.

(*d*) Girls have prolonged growth compared to boys.

Answer (*b*).

Puberty and the adolescent growth spurt occur on the average nearly two years earlier in girls than boys. However early maturing boys will reach puberty ahead of slow maturing girls and it must be remembered that chronologic age has very little to do with where an individual stands developmentally.

23. Adenoid facies is a characteristic finding in children with:

(*a*) thumbsucking habit

(*b*) mouth breathing habit

(*c*) tongue thrusting habit

(*d*) lip biting habit

Answer (*b*).

Adenoid facies is a characteristic finding in children with mouth breathing habit. Mouth breathing is mostly due to nasal airway obstruction. Two locations that have been suggested consistently as sites of nasal obstruction are the nasal turbinates and the nasopharyngeal adenoid tissues. However it does not imply that turbinectomies or adenoidectomies are required to clear the airway.

24. Treatment of choice of habitual mouth breathing is:

(*a*) inclined plane

(*b*) tongue spikes

(*c*) oral screen

(*d*) activator

Answer (*c*).

Oral screen is otherwise called vestibular screen. It is used to correct mouth breathing.

Chapter 18

Diagnosis and Correction of Minor Irregularities in the Developing Dentition

1. Anterior crossbite involving one of the permanent incisors should be corrected:

(*a*) as soon as it is detected

(*b*) at the age of 7 years

(*c*) before the eruption of permanent canines

(*d*) after the eruption of permanent canines

Answer (*a*).

Anterior crossbite of one or more of the permanent incisors should be treated as soon as it is detected. Delayed treatment can lead to serious complications such as loss of arch length, gingival stripping, etc.

2. Delayed treatment of anterior crossbite can lead to:

(*a*) loss of arch length

(*b*) gingival stripping because of traumatic occlusion

(*c*) wear facets on the labial and incisal surfaces of involved incisors

(*d*) any of the above

Answer (*d*).

Delayed treatment of anterior crossbite can lead to any of the above mentioned complications.

3. Anterior crossbite is caused by:

(*a*) presénce of a supernumerary tooth

(*b*) trauma to primary teeth resulting in displacement of permanent teeth

(*c*) an arch length deficiency

(*d*) all of the above

Answer (*d*).

All of the above mentioned causes can lead to anterior crossbite. A labially positioned supernumerary tooth may cause lingual deflection of an incisor, which may erupt in a crossbite relationship. Trauma to primary tooth or delayed exfoliation of primary tooth can lead to displacement of permanent tooth and eruption in crossbite. An arch length deficiency in the maxillary arch can cause the maxillary lateral incisor to erupt palatally resulting in anterior crossbite.

4. Which of the following factors should be present to correct anterior crossbite by simple appliances?

(*a*) Sufficient room should be present mesiodistally to move the tooth into its correct position.

(*b*) Sufficient overbite should be present to hold the tooth in its new position.

(*c*) The apical portion of the in locked tooth should be relatively in the same position as that of the normal tooth.

(*d*) The patient should have normal occlusion in the molar and canine areas.

(*e*) All of the above.

Answer (*e*).

If all of the above mentioned factors are present, then the case may be considered uncomplicated and anterior crossbite can be corrected with simple appliances.

5. Teeth in the initial stage of eruption with a minimal degree of interlocking (crossbite) can be repositioned within 24 hours with:

(*a*) lower cemented bite plane

(*b*) tongue blade therapy

(*c*) appliance with double cantilever spring

(*d*) fixed appliance

Answer (*b*).

In children who are cooperative and have proper encouragement and guidance at home, an anterior crossbite (developing crossbite) can be corrected with a narrow wooden tongue blade. The child is instructed to place the tongue blade behind the inlocked tooth and use the chin as fulcrum to exert pressure on the tooth towards the labial side. This procedure should be practiced at least 5 minutes each hour as often as possible during the day. But the results of this therapy are often disappointing because of lack of cooperation. Lower cemented bite plane (inclined plane) is indicated when the posterior teeth are not present for retention for removable Hawley's appliance with double cantilever spring.

A removable Hawley's appliance with double cantilever spring is the widely used treatment option to correct anterior crossbite. Fixed appliance is used to correct anterior crossbite when adequate space is not available for the tooth to move in a labial position (Severe arch length deficiency).

6. Which of the following is true about tongue blade therapy?

(*a*) The tongue blade is used, using the chin as fulcrum and exerting pressure on the tooth towards the labial side.

(*b*) The procedure should be practiced at least 5 minutes every hour during the day.

(*c*) It is used to correct the teeth in the initial stage of eruption with minimal degree of interlocking.

(*d*) All of the above.

Answer (*d*).

All of the above mentioned factors are true regarding tongue blade therapy.

7. Which of the following is true regarding the inclined plane?

(*a*) The inclination of the inclined plane is 45 degrees to the long axis of the lower incisors.

(*b*) After placing the inclined plane, the posterior teeth should be out of contact by 2–3 mm.

(*c*) Patient should be seen every 2–3 days.

(*d*) All of the above.

Answer (*d*).

All of the above mentioned factors are true regarding inclined plane. Also the child should be encouraged to follow a normal diet and the physical activities should be restricted.

8. W-arch (Porter appliance) and Quadhelix appliances are used for crossbite correction. A fixed acrylic jackscrew appliance causes palatal expansion and less dental tipping.

(*a*) Both the statements are false.

(*b*) Both the statements are true.

(*c*) First statement is true and the second is false.

(*d*) First statement is false and the second is true.

Answer (*b*).

The soldered W-arch or Porter appliance is an efficient appliance for correction of posterior crossbite. This may sometimes function as a reminder appliance in some cases of posterior crossbite associated with thumbsucking.

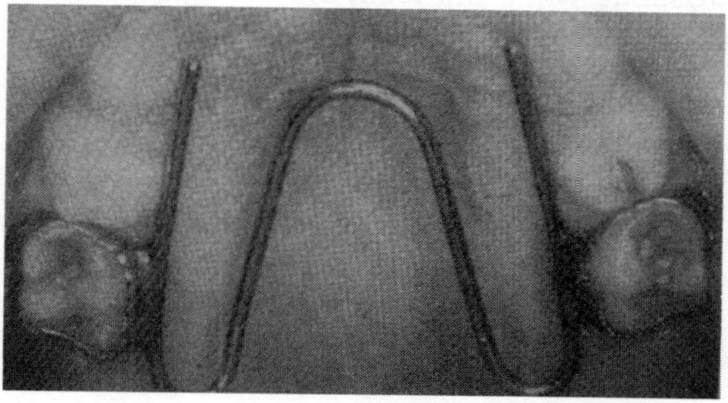

Fig. 18.1 Soldered W-arch for maxillary expansion.

9. A low tongue position can result in the application of unequal forces to the maxillary posterior teeth and can allow these teeth to assume crossbite relationship with

mandibular teeth. In patients who breathe through their mouths the tongue can assume a low position in the mouth resulting in muscle imbalance and subsequently a buccal crossbite.

(*a*) Both the statements are false.

(*b*) Both the statements are true.

(*c*) First statement is true and the second is false.

(*d*) First statement is false and the second is true.

Answer (*b*).

The answer is self-explanatory.

10. A functional crossbite results from the mandible shifting into an abnormal but often more comfortable position. If there is no evidence of a discrepancy in the upper and lower midline when the mandible is at rest, but there is a deviation of the mandible towards the side of the crossbite when the teeth are brought into occlusion, the malocclusion is considered functional.

(*a*) Both the statements are false.

(*b*) Both the statements are true.

(*c*) First statement is true and the second is false.

(*d*) First statement is false and the second is true.

Answer (*b*).

The answer is self-explanatory.

11. If the first permanent molar (only) is in crossbite in one of the sides, the method of choice for correction of posterior crossbite is:

(*a*) W-soldered arch

(*b*) quadhelix appliance

(*c*) cross elastic technique

(*d*) expansion appliance with jackscrew

Answer (*c*).

When the posterior crossbite is involves a single tooth, the treatment of choice is cross elastics. Normally the correction can be achieved in 4–8 weeks with this technique.

12. Ectopic eruption of first permanent molars is more common in the mandible. It is more frequently observed in girls than boys.

(*a*) Both the statements are false.

(*b*) Both the statements are true.

(*c*) First statement is true and the second is false.

(*d*) First statement is false and the second is true.

Answer (*a*).

The reverse is true. Ectopic eruption of first permanent molars is more common in the maxilla. It is more frequently observed in boys than girls.

13. Ectopic eruption of first permanent molars can be corrected by:

(*a*) helical spring (*b*) open coil spring

(*c*) brass ligature wire (*d*) any of the above

Answer (*d*).

Ectopic eruption can be corrected by any of the above mentioned treatment options.

14. At what age is the child expected to have 12 primary teeth and 12 erupted permanent teeth?

(*a*) 5 years (*b*) 7 years

(*c*) 9 years (*d*) 12 years

Answer (*c*).

At 9 years the primary canines, first and second primary molars are usually present. This in each quadrant represents the 12 primary teeth. In permanent teeth the first molars, central and lateral incisors are present at 9 years, which is totally 12 permanent teeth.

15. Serial extraction is referred (Dewel) to as orderly removal of selected primary and permanent teeth in a predetermined sequence. Serial extraction is indicated primarily in severe class I malocclusion in the mixed dentition that has insufficient arch length for the amount of tooth material.

(*a*) Both the statements are false.

(*b*) Both the statements are true.

(*c*) First statement is true and the second is false.

(*d*) First statement is false and the second is true.

Answer (*b*).

The answer is self-explanatory.

16. Which of the following is not true of "mature swallow"?

(*a*) Relaxation of lips.

(*b*) Placement of tongue behind maxillary incisors.

(*c*) Elevation of mandible.

(*d*) This usually occurs before three years of age.

Answer (*d*).

Relaxation of lips, placement of tongue behind maxillary incisors and elevation of mandible is characteristics of mature swallow. However, this pattern of swallowing is not established before 3 years of age.

17. Dental arch circumference reduces during:

(*a*) primary dentition period

(*b*) late transition period

(*c*) permanent dentition period

(*d*) both (*b*) and (*c*).

Answer (*d*).

In late transition period due to the early and late mesial shift, reduction of the arch length occurs. In permanent dentition, continuous proximal wear results in reduction in arch length.

18. Which of the following factors contribute to accommodation of larger permanent incisors?

(*a*) Presence of interdental spaces in the primary anterior teeth.

(*b*) The more labial placement of the crowns increasing the arch circumference.

(*c*) Increase in intercanine diameter.

(*d*) All of the above.

Answer (*d*).

All of the above mentioned factors contribute to the larger permanent incisors. This is known as incisal liability.

19. Maximum intercanine width in mandible is completed by:

(*a*) 4–5 years
(*b*) 7–8 years
(*c*) 9–10 years
(*d*) 10–12 years

Answer (*c*).

The answer is self-explanatory.

Chapter 19

Space Management

1. Which of the following consideration is important to a dentist when space maintenance is considered?

(*a*) Time elapsed since loss of tooth.

(*b*) Amount of bone covering the unerupted tooth.

(*c*) Dental age of the patient.

(*d*) All of the above.

Answer (*d*).

All of the above mentioned factors have to be evaluated while considering space maintenance. Premature loss of primary teeth can lead to space loss in the arches. If space loss occurs, it usually takes place during the first six months after the extraction. It is wise to insert a space maintainer as soon as the tooth is lost. Erupting premolars usually require 4–5 months to move through 1 mm of bone. Hence bone covering the unerupted permanent tooth has to be assessed before placing a space maintainer. Studies by Gron have indicated that the loss of primary molar before 7 years of age (chronologic) will lead to delayed eruption of succedaneous tooth, whereas the loss after 7 years of age leads to an early emergence.

2. Primate spaces are present:

(*a*) mesial to maxillary canines and distal to mandibular canines

(*b*) mesial to mandibular canines and distal to maxillary canines

(*c*) mesial to maxillary and mandibular canines

(*d*) distal to maxillary and mandibular canines

Answer (*a*).

Primate spaces are present mesial to maxillary canines and distal to mandibular canines. They are known as simian spaces or anthropoid spaces.

3. Primate spaces are otherwise called:

(*a*) simian spaces

(*b*) primate spaces by Baume

(*c*) anthropoid spaces

(*d*) all of the above

Answer (*d*).

All of the above mentioned names are used alternatively to denote primate spaces. Baume first reported this in 1950.

4. Flush terminal plane refers to:

(*a*) primary cuspids

(*b*) first permanent molars

(*c*) permanent second molars

(*d*) second primary molars

Answer (*d*).

When the distal surfaces of second primary molars are in a straight line, it is referred to as flush terminal plane. When the distal surface of the lower second primary molar is mesial to the same surface of the maxillary molar it is known as mesial step. In distal step, the distal surface of the lower second primary molar is distal to the same surface of the maxillary molar.

5. Spaces between anterior primary teeth are:

(*a*) uncommon and undesirable

(*b*) common and undesirable

(*c*) common and desirable

(*d*) uncommon and desirable

Answer (*c*).

Spacing between primary anterior teeth is commonly seen and desirable. This is known as physiological spacing. These spaces help the larger sized permanent teeth to erupt in normal alignment. Whenever these spaces are not present in primary dentition, it results in crowding of the permanent dentition.

6. Which of the following is not an example of unilateral fixed space maintainer?

(*a*) Distal shoe

(*b*) Band and loop

(*c*) Nance arch

(*d*) Crown and loop

Answer (*c*).

Nance arch is a bilateral fixed space maintainer indicated when there is bilateral tooth loss in the maxilla. Distal shoe, band and loop and crown and loop are all examples of unilateral fixed space maintainers. Distal shoe is a unilateral fixed space maintainer used when the primary second molar is lost prematurely before the eruption of first permanent molar. Band and loop is a unilateral fixed space maintainer used when there is premature loss of primary molar in one side of the arch. Crown and loop is a unilateral fixed space maintainer indicated when there is unilateral tooth loss. Usually crown and loop is preferred over band and loop when the abutment tooth had pulp treatment (pulpotomy or pulpectomy) before.

Classification of space maintainers and few examples

Fixed	Band and loop
Removable	Acrylic partial denture
Unilateral	Crown and loop
Bilateral	Nance arch, Lingual arch
Active	Wilson arch
Passive	Band and loop
Functional	Acrylic partial denture
Non-functional	Band and loop

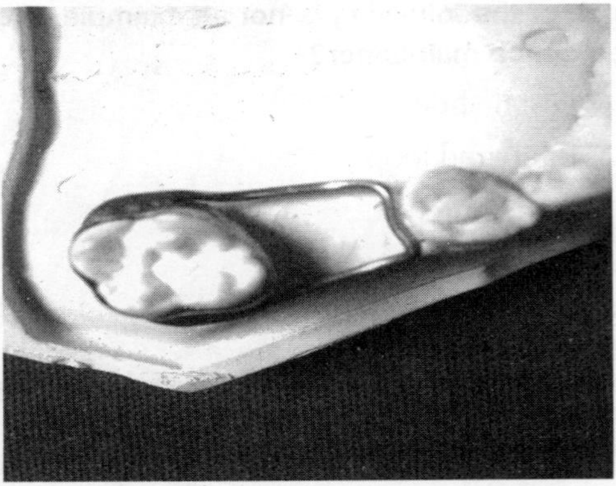

Fig. 19.1 Band and loop space maintainer.

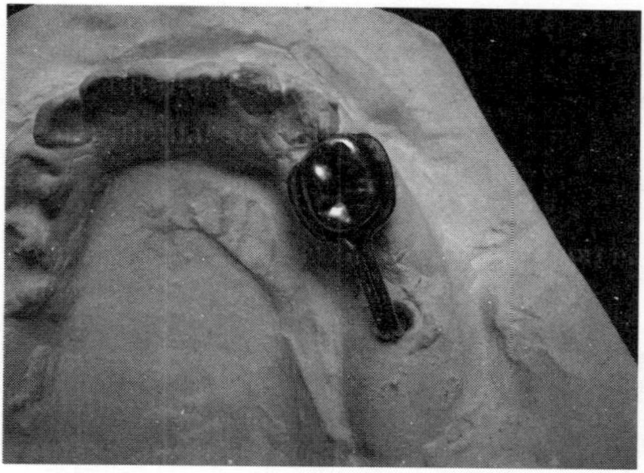

Fig. 19.2 Distal shoe space maintainer.

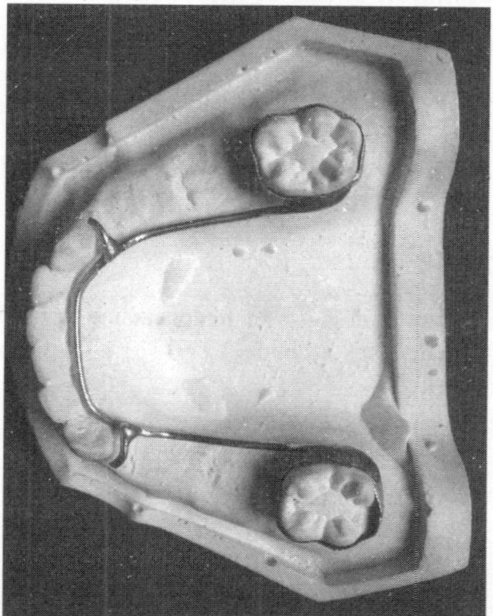

Fig. 19.3 Lingual arch space maintainer.

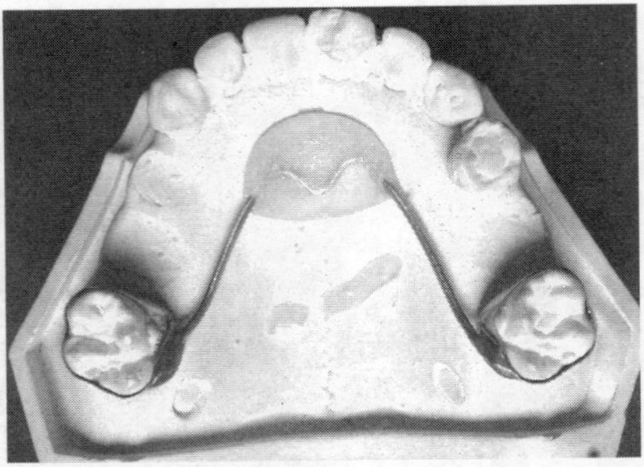

Fig. 19.4 Nance palatal arch space maintainer.

7. Most common cause of malocclusion is:

(*a*) hypothyroidism

(*b*) presence of supernumerary tooth

(*c*) early loss of primary teeth

(*d*) congenital absence of third molars

Answer (*c*).

The most common cause of malocclusion is premature loss of primary teeth. This amounts to 60–70% of the malalignments encountered.

8. Early mesial shift utilizes:

(*a*) leeway space of Nance

(*b*) primate spaces

(*c*) Meyer's space

(*d*) von Ebner's space

Answer (*b*).

Primate spaces are spaces present mesial to the maxillary canines and distal to the mandibular canines. They are used for early mesial shift. There is no space called Meyer's or von Ebner's space.

Leeway space of Nance—the combined mesiodistal width of primary canines, first and second molars is greater than the combined mesiodistal width of unerupted permanent canines and premolars. The difference in the maxilla is 1.8 mm and in the mandible is 3.4 mm (both the sides). This space is utilized by late mesial shift to achieve Class I molar relationship when the primary teeth do not have primate spaces.

9. Late mesial shift utilizes:

(*a*) leeway space of Nance

(*b*) primate spaces

(*c*) Meyer's space

(*d*) von Ebner's space

Answer (*a*).

Refer to the explanation of Q. No. 8.

10. According to Nance, the average amount of leeway space present in the maxillary arch is:

(*a*) 1.8 mm (*b*) 0.9 mm

(*c*) 1.7 mm (*d*) 3.4 mm

Answer (*a*).

The amount of leeway space present in the maxilla is 0.9 mm on either side. Hence the total leeway space present in the maxilla is 1.8 mm.

11. A distal step relationship of the second primary molars is indicative of:

(*a*) Class I malocclusion

(*b*) Class II malocclusion

(*c*) Class III malocclusion

(*d*) Class II div. I

Answer (*b*).

In distal-step relationship, the distal surface of the mandibular second primary molar is distal to the maxillary second molar. This results in the eruption of maxillary first permanent molar mesial to the mandibular first permanent molar resulting in a class II molar relationship.

Mesial step First permanent molar erupts in class I molar relationship (mandibular second molar mesial to maxillary second molar).

Distal step First permanent molar erupts in class II molar relationship.

Flush terminal plane (with primate spaces) First permanent molar erupts in end on relationship. Class I molar relationship is achieved by early mesial shift.

Flush terminal plane (without primate spaces) First permanent molar erupts in end on relationship. Class I molar relationship is achieved by late mesial shift.

12. Advantage of Moyer's mixed dentition analysis over Nance is:

(*a*) it can be performed only in the maxillary arch

(*b*) it does not require a radiograph

(*c*) it can be done before the eruption of permanent incisors

(*d*) it can be performed in the primary dentition itself

Answer (*b*).

Moyer's mixed dentition analysis uses a probability chart and does not need a radiograph. This can be performed both in the maxilla and the mandible. To perform a mixed dentition analysis mandibular permanent incisors must be present. Moyer, Nance, and Tanaka-Johnson analysis uses the mesiodistal width of mandibular permanent incisors as standards. All the mixed dentition analyses uses mesiodistal width of mandibular permanent incisors as standards because of their early eruption and less susceptibility for morphological variations. It cannot be performed in primary dentition because of the absence of mandibular permanent incisors.

13. While using Moyer's probability chart the percentage level of probability used for space prediction is:

(*a*) 25%

(*b*) 50%

(*c*) 75%

(*d*) 100%

Answer (*c*).

The percentage level used for space prediction using Moyer's probability chart is 75%.

14. In Tanaka-Johnson analysis the value that is added for prediction of required space in maxillary arch is:

(*a*) 11

(*b*) 10.5

(*c*) 12

(*d*) 9.5

Answer (*a*).

The formula used for space prediction in Tanaka-Johnson analysis is as follows.

(*a*) **In maxilla**

$$\frac{\text{Combined mesiodistal width of mandibular central and lateral incisors} + 11}{2}$$

(*b*) **In mandible**

$$\frac{\text{Combined mesiodistal width of mandibular central and lateral incisors} + 10.5}{2}$$

15. A 4-year-old child who has to undergo removal of severely decayed second primary molar would require a:

(*a*) band and loop space maintainer

(*b*) crown and loop space maintainer

(*c*) distal shoe space maintainer

(*d*) reverse band and loop space maintainer

Answer (*c*).

As the first permanent molars would not have erupted by then, the space maintainer indicated in this situation is distal shoe space maintainer. It will guide the eruption of first permanent molar. Refer to the explanation of Q. No. 6.

16. An 8-year-old patient who has lost all the four maxillary primary molars would require:

(*a*) Nance arch space maintainer

(*b*) lingual arch space maintainer

(*c*) passive lingual arch space maintainer

(*d*) band and loop

Answer (*a*).

Nance arch space maintainer is indicated when there is premature bilateral loss of primary molars in the maxilla. In a similar situation in the mandible the choice of space maintainer will be passive lingual arch. On the other hand, band and loop space maintainer is indicated when there is unilateral loss of primary tooth either in the mandible or in the maxilla.

17. A 6-year-old child who has lost all the four mandibular primary molars (lower permanent incisors have not erupted) and the permanent first molars are partially erupted, would require a:

(*a*) Nance arch space maintainer

(*b*) lingual arch space maintainer

(*c*) removable acrylic partial denture

(*d*) band and loop

Answer (*c*).

Presence of mandibular permanent incisors is a prerequisite for a lingual arch space maintainer as the lingual arch rests on the cingulum of permanent incisors. As the lower permanent molars are partially erupted, banding of these teeth for a lingual arch is not possible. Nance arch space maintainer is used in the maxilla and band and loop space maintainer in unilateral tooth loss situations. Therefore removable of partial denture (as a functional type) is the treatment of choice.

18. In a 6-year-old child who has lost mandibular right first primary molar and has an endodontically treated second primary molar, the space maintainer of choice will be:

(*a*) band and loop

(*b*) crown and loop

(*c*) lingual arch

(*d*) reverse crown and loop

Answer (*b*).

As the endodontically treated mandibular second molar can serve as an abutment, crown and loop space maintainer will be the treatment of choice. Reverse crown and loop space maintainer is indicated when the second primary molar is lost after the eruption of first permanent molar (partially erupted) in which the first primary molar is endodontically treated.

19. All of the following are examples of nonfunctional space maintainer except:

(*a*) band and loop

(*b*) crown and loop

(*c*) acrylic partial denture

(*d*) lingual arch

Answer (*c*).

Space maintainers that have components participating in mastication are called functional space maintainers. In other words the space maintainer should replace the function of the tooth, which is lost prematurely. Of the space maintainers mentioned above, only the acrylic partial denture can have teeth on it, which can help the patient chew.

20. One of the following space maintainer is otherwise called eruption-guiding appliance:

(*a*) band and loop

(*b*) crown and loop

(*c*) distal shoe

(*d*) reverse crown and loop

Answer (*c*).

Distal shoe space maintainer is otherwise called eruption guiding appliance and intra-alveolar appliance because the intra-alveolar extension of the distal shoe space maintainer guides the eruption of unerupted first permanent molar.

21. Major disadvantage of removable space maintainer is that it:

(*a*) is difficult to keep it clean

(*b*) cannot be made esthetic

(*c*) will not maintain the vertical dimension

(*d*) may not be worn

Answer (*d*).

The major drawback of a removable space maintainer is that the patient may not wear it consistently.

22. The treatment of choice for a normal girl whose dental age is 10 years and who has lost a mandibular primary first molar unilaterally would be:

(*a*) a stainless steel crown and a loop space maintainer

(*b*) an acrylic unilateral partial denture

(*c*) a band and loop space maintainer

(*d*) no treatment required

Answer (*d*).

As the patient's dental age is 10 years the first premolar should erupt soon. Hence, there is no need for a space maintainer.

23. An 8-year-old patient has an end on molar relation and normal vertical and horizontal overlap. The mandibular lateral incisors are erupting slightly lingually. The dentist should:

(*a*) insert a lingual arch
(*b*) refer him to an orthodontist
(*c*) continue routine dental care and developmental supervision
(*d*) institute orthodontic therapy to reposition the lateral incisors to correct the Class II molar relationship

Answer (*c*).

As the mandibular incisors are erupting lingually the patient should be under developmental supervision, as he may need serial extraction or proximal stripping in due course of time.

24. In a mixed dentition space analysis, the most careful estimate will only be accurate within:

(*a*) 0.5 mm
(*b*) 2 mm
(*c*) 4 mm
(*d*) 6 mm

Answer (*b*).

Among the existing mixed dentition space analysis the most careful estimate will be accurate within 2 mm.

25. The band and loop space maintainer is classified as:

(*a*) bilateral, fixed, functional
(*b*) unilateral, fixed, functional
(*c*) unilateral, fixed and nonfunctional
(*d*) unilateral, removable and nonfunctional

Answer (*c*).

The answer is self-explanatory. Refer to the explanation of Q. No. 19.

26. Space maintainer is least indicated for premature loss of:

(*a*) primary maxillary first molar

(*b*) primary mandibular first molar

(*c*) primary maxillary central incisor

(*d*) permanent maxillary central incisor

Answer (*c*).

Premature loss of primary anterior teeth does not cause space loss whereas traumatic loss of permanent anterior teeth causes space loss. Also premature loss of primary molars causes space loss.

27. A mixed dentition analysis determines:

(*a*) inter canine width

(*b*) skeletal growth pattern

(*c*) discrepancies in jaw size

(*d*) space available versus space required

Answer (*d*).

In a mixed dentition analysis the permanent mandibular anterior teeth are used as standards for prediction of the sizes of unerupted permanent teeth. This gives the space available and the space required.

28. When dealing with decayed primary teeth the best space maintainer is a:

(*a*) lingual arch

(*b*) band and loop

(*c*) properly restored primary tooth

(*d*) functional removable space maintainer

Answer (*c*).

Natural teeth are the best space maintainers. Hence a properly restored primary tooth is the best space maintainer of all.

Chapter 20

Management of Disabled and Medically Compromised Children

1. In which of the following clinical situation the dietary intake of the child has restriction of specific foods or total caloric consumption:

(*a*) phenylketonuria

(*b*) diabetes

(*c*) prader-Willi syndrome

(*d*) all of the above

Answer (*d*).

Patients with metabolic disturbances or syndromes like Phenylketonuria, Diabetes and Prader-Willi syndrome have diets that restrict specific foods or caloric consumption. The dietary recommendations should be made individually after proper consultation with the patient's primary physician or dietician.

2. Which of the following is not an indication for the use of physical restraints?

(*a*) A patient who requires diagnosis or treatment and cannot cooperate because of lack of maturity

(*b*) A patient who requires diagnosis or treatment and cannot cooperate because of mental or physical disabilities

(*c*) A patient who requires diagnosis or treatment and does not cooperate and other behaviour management techniques have failed

(*d*) When the safety of the patient or the practitioner would be at risk without the protective use of restraint

Answer (*c*).

Choice 'c' is not an indication for physical restraint. Physical restraint should be used in a patient who requires diagnosis or treatment and does not cooperate only after the other behaviour management techniques have failed. All the other choices are indications for using physical restraint.

3. Which of the following is not an aid in maintaining the mouth in an open position?

(*a*) Padded tongue blade

(*b*) Molt mouth prop

(*c*) McKesson mouth prop

(*d*) Towel and tape

Answer (*d*).

Common mechanical aids for maintaining the mouth in open position are wrapped tongue blades, open wide disposable mouth props, molt mouth prop and McKesson bite-blocks. Padded and wrapped tongue blades are easy to use, disposable and inexpensive. Open wide mouth props are also easy to use but are slightly more expensive than the wrapped blades. They are available in two sizes. Molt mouth prop is used in the management of difficult patients for prolonged periods. It is available in adult and child sizes and it gives accessibility to the opposite side of the mouth. It has the disadvantage of causing lip and palatal ulcerations and luxation of teeth if not used correctly. Rubber bite blocks available in various sizes can be used to stabilize the mouth in the open position. Always remember that the patient's mouth should not be forcibly stretched because it may cause further resistance and airway compromise.

4. Which of the following physical restraints is not used to control body position?

(*a*) Papoose board (*b*) Pedi wrap

(*c*) Safety belt (*d*) Posey straps

Answer (*d*).

Refer to the table below:

S. No.	***Body part***	***Restraints***
1.	Body	Papoose board Triangular sheet Pedi wrap Beanbag dental chair insert Safety belt Extra assistant
2.	Extremities	Posey straps Velcro straps Towel and tape Extra assistant
3.	Head	Forearm body support Head positioner Plastic bowl Extra assistant

Posey straps are used to control extremities whereas all the other three are used to control body position on the dental chair. The Papoose board is available in different sizes to hold large and small children. It is simple to use and store and has attached head stabilizers. An extremely resistant patient may develop hyperthermia if immobilized for too long. The pedi wrap does not have head straps or back board. It is made up of mesh fabric which permits better ventilation and lessens the chances of hyperthermia. The bean bag dental chair insert comfortably accommodates hypotonic and spastic children who need more support and less immobilization. It actually encourages relaxation and allows the dental work to be done more efficiently.

5. All of the following physical restraints are used to control extremities except:

(*a*) posey straps (*b*) velcro straps

(*c*) towel and tape (*d*) triangular sheet

Answer (*d*).

Triangular sheet is not used to restrict the extremities. The child's arms and legs can be immobilized with posey straps, a towel and adhesive tape, velcro straps or with the help of an extra assistant. Refer to the explanation of Q. No. 4.

6. Which of the following restraints was developed to help comfortably accommodate the hypotonic and severely spastic persons?

(*a*) Bean bag dental chair insert.

(*b*) Pedi wrap.

(*c*) Papoose board.

(*d*) Posey straps.

Answer (*a*).

The beanbag dental insert was developed to help comfortable accommodation of the hypotonic and severely spastic persons as they need more support and less immobilization on a dental chair. They also relax in this type of setting.

7. Which of the medical conditions increase the mortality of infants and children with Down syndrome?

(*a*) Cardiac defects.

(*b*) Increased incidence of leukemia.

(*c*) Increased incidence of upper respiratory infections.

(*d*) All of the above.

Answer (*d*).

All of the above mentioned medical conditions are responsible for increased mortality of infants and children with Down's syndrome or Trisomy 21. The incidence of cardiac defects is about 40%. These children also have a ten to twenty fold increase in the incidence of leukemia when compared to the general population. There is also a high incidence of rapid destructive periodontal disease noticed in these children.

8. Fragile X syndrome is a common inherited form of mental retardation and autism. It accounts for 30% to 50% of cases of X-linked mental retardation.

(*a*) Both the statements are true.

(*b*) Both the statements are false.

(*c*) The first statement is true and the second is false.

(*d*) The first statement is false and the second is true.

Answer (*a*).

The answer is self-explanatory. The defect in this syndrome is the presence of an abnormal gene on the terminal portion of the long arm of X chromosome. Males are more vulnerable as they have only one X chromosome and are also more significantly affected than females.

9. In which of the following conditions is there a high incidence of dental and skeletal malocclusions?

(*a*) Prader-Willi syndrome.

(*b*) Fragile X syndrome.

(*c*) Fetal Alcohol Syndrome.

(*d*) Autism.

Answer (*c*).

Most of the dental problems associated with FAS (Fetal Alcohol Syndrome) children are related to the high incidence of dental and skeletal malocclusions. The consumption of 1 to 3 drinks per day during the first two months of pregnancy can result in significant damage to the developing baby. Other complications in such babies include neurologic abnormalities, cardiac defects, growth retardation and cognitive defects.

10. Autism is a severely incapacitating disturbance of mental and emotional development that causes problems in learning, communication, and relating to others. This lifelong developmental disability which manifests itself during the first three years of life is difficult to diagnose and has no cure.

(*a*) Both the statements are true.

(*b*) Both the statements are false.

(*c*) The first statement is true and the second is false.

(*d*) The first statement is false and the second is true.

Answer (*a*).

The answer is self-explanatory. Autism occurs approximately in five out of every 10,000 births and is more common in boys. These children have multiple medical and behavioural problems, which make their dental treatment difficult.

11. Which of the following is true of autism?

(*a*) Autistic children look like normal children and have normal lifespans but they have limited capacity to communicate, socialize and learn.

(*b*) Autistic children have poor muscle tone, poor coordination, drooling, a hyperactive knee jerk, strabismus and some children eventually develop epilepsy.

(*c*) Autistic children have strict routines and prefer soft and sweetened foods. Because of poor tongue coordination they tend to pouch food instead of swallowing.

(*d*) All of the above.

Answer (*d*).

All the above statements regarding autism are true. These children apart from having a tendency to pouch food instead of swallowing also have an increased desire for sweets. This leads to increased to caries susceptibility.

12. The disability involved in patients with cerebral palsy can be:

(*a*) muscle weakness

(*b*) paralysis or stiffness

(*c*) poor balance or irregular gait

(*d*) uncoordinated or involuntary movements

(*e*) Any of the above

Answer (*e*).

Cerebral palsy is one of the primary handicapping conditions of childhood with an incidence of 1 in 200 live births approximately. The disability in these children includes any of the four choices above.

13. Cerebral palsy is classified based on the neuromuscular dysfunction and the extent of anatomic involvement. The cause for one third of cerebral palsy cases is not known.

(*a*) Both the statements are true.

(*b*) Both the statements are false.

(*c*) The first statement is true and the second is false.

(*d*) The first statement is false and the second is true.

Answer (*a*).

The answer is self-explanatory.

14. The most common type of cerebral palsy is:

(*a*) dyskinetic (*b*) ataxic

(*c*) spastic (*d*) mixed

Answer (*c*).

The most common type is the spastic type (approximately 70% of cases).

S. No.	*Type*	*% of cases (approximately)*
1.	Spastic	70%
2.	Dyskinetic	15%
3.	Ataxic	5%
4.	Mixed	10%

15. Athetosis and Choreoathetosis are seen in ________ type of cerebral palsy:

(*a*) dyskinetic

(*b*) ataxic

(*c*) spastic

(*d*) mixed

Answer (*a*).

A succession of slow, twisting or writhing involuntary movements (athetosis) or quick jerky movements (choreoathetosis) are features of dyskinetic type of cerebral palsy.

16. Bruxism is most commonly seen in—type of cerebral palsy:

(*a*) dyskinetic

(*b*) ataxic

(*c*) spastic

(*d*) mixed

Answer (*a*).

Bruxism is most commonly seen in dyskinetic type of cerebral palsy. Severe occlusal attrition of the primary and permanent dentition is noticed. T.M. joint disorders may be a sequelae of this condition noticed in adult patients.

17. Limping gait and circumduction of affected leg is characteristic feature in:

(*a*) hemiplegia

(*b*) quadriplegia

(*c*) monoplegia

(*d*) paraplegia

Answer (*a*).

In spastic hemiplegia, the hand and arm are flexed and held against the trunk. The foot and leg may be flexed and rotated internally resulting in a limping gait with circumduction of the affected leg.

S. No.	*Type*	*Description*
1.	Monoplegia	Involvement of one limb only
2.	Hemiplegia	Involvement of one side of the body
3.	Paraplegia	Involvement of both legs only
4.	Diplegia	Involvement of both legs with minimum involvement of both arms
5.	Quadriplegia	Involvement of all four limbs

18. Some of the neonatal reflexes persist long after the age at which they normally disappear in cerebral palsy patients. Which of the following reflexes is retained?

(*a*) Asymmetric tonic neck reflex.

(*b*) Tonic labyrinthine reflex.

(*c*) Startle reflex.

(*d*) All of the above.

Answer (*d*).

In patients with cerebral palsy certain neonatal reflexes may persist long after the age at which they normally disappear. These primitive reflexes are usually modified or are progressively replaced as the subcortical dominance of the infant's behaviour is suppressed by the higher centres of the maturing central nervous system. Three such reflexes are mentioned above.

S. No.	Type	Description
1.	Asymmetric tonic neck reflex	If the patient's head is suddenly turned to one side, the arm and leg on the side to which the face is turned will extend and stiffen. The limbs on the opposite side will flex.
2.	Tonic labyrinthine reflex	If the patient's head suddenly falls backwards while the patient is supine, the back may assume the position known as postural extension; the legs and arms will straighten out and the neck and back will arch.
3.	Startle reflex	Sudden, involuntary and forceful bodily movements are produced when the patient is surprised by stimuli such as sudden noises or unexpected movements by other people.

19. If a patient's (cerebral palsy) head suddenly falls backward while the patient is in a supine position, legs and arms straighten out and the neck and back will arch. Which reflex is this?

(*a*) Asymmetric tonic neck reflex.

(*b*) Tonic labyrinthine reflex.

(*c*) Startle reflex.

(*d*) All of the above.

Answer (*b*).

Refer to the explanation of Q. No. 18.

20. Which of the following is considered as one of the approaches in handling children with cerebral palsy in the dental office?

(*a*) Providing dental treatment in the wheel chair.

(*b*) Use of mouth props and finger splints.

(*c*) Avoidance of abrupt stimuli which will initiate the startle reflex.

(*d*) All of the above.

Answer (*d*).

All the above approaches are to be used while handling a child with cerebral palsy in the dental office.

21. Difficulty in grasping objects is characteristic of which type of cerebral palsy:

(*a*) dyskinetic (*b*) ataxic

(*c*) spastic (*d*) mixed

Answer (*b*).

Poor sense of balance and uncoordinated voluntary movements (e.g. stumbling or staggering gait or difficulty in grasping objects) is characteristic of ataxic type of cerebral palsy.

22. The touch taste smell method (instead of TSD) is usually used in children who are affected by:

(*a*) deafness (*b*) blindness

(*c*) cerebral palsy (*d*) Down's syndrome

Answer (*b*).

The touch taste smell method is used in children affected with blindness, as these senses are acute in these children.

23. Which of the following factors are to be considered while treating a child whose hearing is impaired?

(*a*) Determining the mode of communication.

(*b*) Usage of visual aids and allows the patient to see the instruments.

(*c*) Adjusting the hearing aids.

(*d*) All of the above.

Answer (*d*).

All the above factors must be considered while treating a child whose hearing is impaired.

24. Which of the following factors are to be considered while treating a child who is blind?

(*a*) Reassuring physical contact.

(*b*) Detailed description of the office and the instruments to be used.

(*c*) Do not move, grab or stop the patient without verbal warning.

(*d*) Usage of audio cassettes and Braille pamphlets.

(*e*) All of the above.

Answer (*e*).

All the above factors are to be considered while treating a child who is blind. Making physical contact like holding the patient's hand often promotes relaxation.

25. In a patient with cardiac disease (susceptible to infective endocarditis) pulp therapy of primary teeth is not recommended. In permanent dentition endodontic therapy may be undertaken after a careful evaluation and case selection.

(*a*) Both the statements are true.

(*b*) Both the statements are false.

(*c*) The first statement is true and the second is false.

(*d*) The first statement is false and the second is true.

Answer (*a*).

Pulp therapy for primary teeth with poor prognosis is not recommended because of the high incidence of associated chronic infection. Extraction of such teeth and appropriate fixed space maintainers are preferred. Endodontic therapy in the permanent dentition can usually be accomplished successfully if the teeth are carefully selected and endodontic therapy is adequately performed.

26. Rheumatic fever is common in which of the following age groups:

(*a*) less than 6 years

(*b*) 6–15 years

(*c*) 15–30 years

(*d*) more than 30 years

Answer (*b*).

Rheumatic fever appears most commonly between 6–15 years of age. It is rare in infancy. It is most prevalent in temperate zones, high altitudes and is more common and severe in children who live in substandard conditions.

27. The acute form of bacterial endocarditis is a fulminating disease that usually occurs as a result of micro-organisms of high pathogenicity attacking a normal heart, causing erosive destruction of valves. Subacute bacterial endocarditis usually develops in a person with pre-existing congenital cardiac disease or rheumatic valvular lesions.

(*a*) Both the statements are true.

(*b*) Both the statements are false.

(*c*) The first statement is true and the second is false.

(*d*) The first statement is false and the second is true.

Answer (*a*).

The acute form is caused by Staphylococcus, Group A Streptococcus and Pneumococcus whereas the subacute form is caused by Streptococci viridans.

28. Which of the following is correct regarding the agent and dosage used for antibiotic prophylaxis?

(*a*) Amoxicillin; adults–2 gm and children 50 mg/kg one hour prior to the procedure.

(*b*) Clindamycin; adults–600 mg and children 20 mg/kg one hour prior to the procedure.

(*c*) Azithromycin or Clarithromycin; adults 500 mg and children 15 mg/kg one hour prior to the procedure.

(*d*) Any of the above.

Answer (*d*).

Any dental patient, who has a history of congenital heart disease or rheumatic heart disease or who has a prosthetic valve should be considered susceptible. With only one large dose of antibiotics, routine restorative and surgical dental procedures, which are known to precipitate transient bacteremia, can be safely completed. All the above regimens can be used as antibiotic prophylaxis for dental, oral, respiratory tract or esophageal procedures.

29. Which of the following factors are correct regarding Hemophilia A?

(*a*) It is caused by a deficiency of factor VIII.

(*b*) It is inherited as X-linked recessive trait.

(*c*) Males are affected and females are carriers.

(*d*) All of the above.

Answer (*d*).

All of the above mentioned factors are correct regarding hemophilia. If a normal male has children with a carrier of hemophilia there is a 50% chance that haemophilia will occur in each male offspring and a 50% chance that each female offspring will be a carrier. If a male hemophilic has children with a normal female, all male offsprings will be normal and all female offsprings will be carriers.

30. Christmas disease is:

(*a*) Hemophilia A

(*b*) Hemophilia B

(*c*) Hemophilia C

(*d*) von Willebrand's disease

Answer (*b*).

Christmas disease is otherwise called hemophilia B. It is caused by deficiency of factor IX (plasma thromboplastin component).

31. Impaired formation of platelet plug in Von Willebrand's disease may result in bleeding from the skin and mucosa, bruising, epistaxis, prolonged bleeding after surgical procedures and menorrhagia. This is in contrast to factors VIII and IX deficient hemophilia in which bleeding tends to involve muscles and joints:

(*a*) both the statements are true

(*b*) both the statements are false

(*c*) the first statement is true and the second is false

(*d*) the first statement is false and the second is true

Answer (*a*).

The answer is self-explanatory.

32. Which of the following agents are used for treatment of hemophilia?

(*a*) Factor VIII concentrate.

(*b*) Synthetic analog of vasopressin (1-deamino-8-D-arginine vasopressin).

(*c*) Epsilon-amino caproic acid.

(*d*) Tranexamic acid.

(*e*) All of the above.

Answer (*e*).

The mainstay of therapy for hemophilia is replacement of coagulation factor either by the use of purified concentrate made from blood plasma or through recombinant technology. DDAVP (1-deamino-8-D-arginine vasopressin) is a synthetic analogue of vasopressin and can be used for minor hemorrhagic episodes to achieve hemostasis. Antifibrinolytics are adjunctive therapies for dental management of patients with bleeding disorders. These agents include epsilon amino caproic acid or tranexamic acid. They prevent the lysis of loose friable clots that a hemophiliac forms within the oral cavity.

33. Periodontal ligament injections are contraindicated in hemophiliac patients. Inferior alveolar nerve block and posterior superior alveolar nerve block predisposes to the development of hematoma, which can lead to airway obstruction.

(*a*) Both the statements are true.

(*b*) Both the statements are false.

(*c*) The first statement is true and the second is false.

(*d*) The first statement is false and the second is true.

Answer (*d*).

In the absence of factor replacement, periodontal ligament (PDL) injections may be used. The anesthetic is administered along the four axial surfaces of the tooth by placement of the needle into the gingival sulcus and the periodontal ligament space. The loose connective, non-fibrous and highly vascularised tissue at the sites of inferior alveolar injection and posterior superior alveolar injections are predisposed to the development of a dissecting hematoma, which has the potential of obstructing the airway and of creating a life-threatening bleeding episode.

34. A pulpotomy or pulpectomy is preferable to extraction in hemophiliac patients. Rubber dam clamp retainers with sub-gingival extensions (8A or 14A) should be avoided.

(*a*) Both the statements are true.

(*b*) Both the statements are false.

(*c*) The first statement is true and the second is false.

(*d*) The first statement is false and the second is true.

Answer (*a*).

The extraction of a tooth in an individual with hemophilia implies more complicated treatment and expense to the patient. Hemorrhage from the pulp chamber does not present a significant problem if readily controlled with pressure from cotton pledgets.

35. Acute hepatitis classically presents with lethargy, loss of appetite, nausea, vomiting, abdominal pain and ultimately jaundice. In children the disease is usually more benign and jaundice is uncommon.

(*a*) Both the statements are true.

(*b*) Both the statements are false.

(*c*) The first statement is true and the second isfalse.

(*d*) The first statement is false and the second is true.

Answer (*a*).

The answer is self-explanatory.

36. The most frequent cause of death in AIDS patients is:

(*a*) Non-Hodgkin's lymphoma

(*b*) Kaposi's sarcoma

(*c*) *Pneumocystis carinii pneumonia*

(*d*) Herpes virus infection

Answer (*c*).

The answer is self-explanatory.

37. The most frequently seen neoplasm in AIDS patients is:

(*a*) Non-Hodgkin's lymphoma

(*b*) Hodgkin's lymphoma

(*c*) Kaposi's sarcoma

(*d*) Burkitt's lymphoma

Answer (*c*).

Often the first lesions of Kaposi sarcoma appear in the oral cavity. The most common oral site is the hard palate. The lesions may be red, blue or purple, flat or raised and solitary or multiple.

38. The leading cause of death in children is:

(*a*) accidents

(*b*) malignancy

(*c*) heart disease

(*d*) respiratory disorders

Answer (*a*).

Malignancy is second only to accidents as the leading cause of death in children.

39. Leukemia is a malignancy of the hematopoietic tissues in which there is a disseminated proliferation of abnormal leukocytes in bone marrow. These immature appearing undifferentiated blast cells replace normal cells in bone marrow and accumulate in other tissues and organs of the body.

(*a*) Both the statements are true.

(*b*) Both the statements are false.

(*c*) The first statement is true and the second is false.

(*d*) The first statement is false and the second is true.

Answer (*a*).

The answer is self-explanatory.

40. The commonest type of leukemia affecting children is:

(*a*) acute lymphocytic leukemia

(*b*) acute myelocytic leukemia

(*c*) chronic lymphocytic leukemia

(*d*) chronic myelocytic leukemia

Answer (*a*).

Acute leukemia is the most common malignancy in children. It accounts for about one-third of all childhood malignancies; of these approximately 80% are lymphocytic (acute lymphocytic leukemia). Chronic leukemia is rare in children accounting for less than 2% of all cases.

41. In a leukemic child whose first remission has not been obtained or one who is in relapse, all elective dental procedures should be deferred. Pulp therapy in primary and permanent teeth are contraindicated in leukemic children.

(*a*) Both the statements are true.

(*b*) Both the statements are false.

(*c*) The first statement is true and the second is false.

(*d*) The first statement is false and the second is true.

Answer (*a*).

Both the statements are true. However, it is essential that potential sources of systemic infection within the oral cavity be controlled or eradicated whenever they are recognized (e.g. immediate extraction of carious primary teeth with pulpal involvement). Endodontic treatment for permanent teeth is not recommended for any patient with leukemia. Even with the most exacting technique, an area of chronic inflammatory tissue may remain in the periapical region, which in an immunosuppressed neutropenic patient can act as an anachoretic focus with devastating sequelae.

42. The minimum platelet level required to perform most dental procedures is:

(*a*) 50,000–100,000/mm^3

(*b*) 200,000–300,000/mm^3

(*c*) 400,000–500,000/mm^3

(*d*) 20,000–50,000/mm^3

Answer (*a*).

A platelet level of 100,000/mm^3 is adequate for most of the dental procedures.

S. No.	*Counts*	*Significance*
1.	1,50,000–400,000	Normal
2.	50,000–100,000	Bleeding time is prolonged, but patient would tolerate most routine procedures
3.	20,000–50,000	At moderate risk of bleeding; defer elective surgery procedures
4.	< 20,000	At significant risk for bleeding; defer elective dental procedures

43. Infection is the primary cause of death in approximately 80% of children with leukemia. Bleeding is the second most common cause.

(*a*) Both the statements are true.

(*b*) Both the statements are false.

(*c*) The first statement is true and the second is false.

(*d*) The first statement is false and the second is true.

Answer (*a*).

The answer is self-explanatory. Hence, the primary objective of dental treatment in a child with leukemia should be the prevention, control and eradication of oral inflammation, hemorrhage and infection.

44. Which of the following disease in children needs bone marrow transplantation?

(*a*) Aplastic anemia.

(*b*) Leukemias.

(*c*) Myelofibrosis.

(*d*) All of the above.

Answer (*d*).

The answer is self-explanatory.

45. The most common cause of failure of bone marrow transplantation is:

(*a*) infection due to endogenous opportunistic microorganisms

(*b*) infection due to extraneous viruses and bacteria

(*c*) post operative hemorrhage

(*d*) any of the above

Answer (*a*).

In almost all organ transplant procedures, host rejection of the transplanted organ and infection are the prime reasons for treatment failure.

46. Which of the following are oral complications of total body irradiation?

(*a*) Mucositis.

(*b*) Transient salivary gland dysfunction.

(*c*) Oral ulceration.

(*d*) Gingival bleeding.

(*e*) Any of the above.

Answer (*e*).

Oral ulceration, mucositis and transient salivary gland dysfunction are frequent consequences of somatotoxic chemotherapy and total body irradiation. Minor trauma to atrophic mucous membranes often results in self-induced ulceration of the buccal mucosa, lips and tongue. Thrombocytopenic gingival bleeding and bleeding from oral ulcerations are also frequently encountered.

47. As a pretransplant preparation which of the following can be undertaken by a patient to maintain good oral hygiene:

(*a*) daily brushing and flossing

(*b*) daily use of self applied topical fluoride gel

(*c*) chlorhexidine mouth rinse every 12 hrs

(*d*) all of the above

Answer (*d*).

The answer is self-explanatory. The integrity of the oral cavity is maintained by keeping the oral structures both hard and soft tissues clean, moist and free of infection. The resultant decrease in septic episodes in the oral cavity should diminish the patient's morbidity and mortality since the mouth is the most common source of infection in these patients.

48. Which of the following malignant diseases is common in childhood?

(*a*) Wilms tumour.

(*b*) Osteosarcoma.

(*c*) Rhabdomyosarcoma.

(*d*) Neuroblastoma.

(*e*) All of the above.

Answer (*e*).

The answer is self-explanatory. Solid tumours account for approximately half of the cases of childhood malignancy. Dental management of patients with solid tumours is similar to that of patients with acute leukemia.

Chapter 21

Genetics and Pediatric Dentistry

1. The genetic material, DNA that controls the production of a single protein (or polypeptide chain) is called a chromosome. There are thousands and thousands of human genes each one regulating the production of a specific polypeptide.

(*a*) Both the statements are true.

(*b*) Both the statements are false.

(*c*) First statement is true and the second is false.

(*d*) First statement is false and the second is true.

Answer (*d*).

Gene is defined as the genetic material that controls the production of a single protein or polypeptide chain. There are thousands of genes, each regulating the production of specific polypeptide. These genes are grouped into units called chromosomes.

2. Who demonstrated the fundamental defect in Down syndrome to be the presence of an extra chromosome in the affected individuals karyotype?

(*a*) Le Jeune (*b*) Turpin

(*c*) Gautier (*d*) All of the above

Answer (*d*).

In 1959 Le Jeune, Turpin and Gautier demonstrated that the fundamental defect in Down syndrome is the presence of an extra chromosome. They have proved this by karyotyping the chromosomes of the affected individuals.

3. Match the following structural alterations of chromosomes:

A	Deletion	1.	The attachment of a broken piece from one chromosome to another non-homologous chromosome.
B	Duplication	2.	The absence of a segment of a chromosome.
C	Inversion	3.	The insertion of an extra fragment into a chromosome from its now deficient homologue.
D	Translocation	4.	The breaking of a chromosome in two places and subsequent rejoining with the middle piece inverted.

(*a*) A-2, B-3, C-4, D-1 (*b*) A-4, B-1, D-2, C-3

(*c*) A-3, B-4, C-1, D-2 (*d*) A-3, B-2, C-1, D-4

Answer (*a*).

Humans have 46 chromosomes. Each chromosome has a pair that is referred to as the homolog. Genes on homologs control the same genetic trait and with the single exception of those genes on the sex chromosomes, there are at least two genes that control each inherited trait

4. Monosomy of an autosome or a missing autosomal chromosome is not believed to be compatible with life.

On the other hand, monosomy of the sex chromosomes does occur and it is compatible with life.

(*a*) Both the statements are true.

(*b*) Both the statements are false.

(*c*) First statement is true and the second is false.

(*d*) First statement is false and the second is true.

Answer (*a*).

In Turner syndrome, monosomy of X chromosome is seen (45 X) and it is compatible with life. But monosomy of an autosome is not compatible with life.

5. All of the following statements are true regarding traits except:

(*a*) monogenic traits are produced and regulated by a single gene.

(*b*) monogenic traits are usually easy to recognize in families and the transmission of the trait from one family member to the next follows simple mendelian principles of dominant recessive, autosomal or sex-linked inheritance.

(*c*) many genes at different loci control polygenic traits.

(*d*) polygenic traits are common and are illustrated by examples such as albinism, achondroplasia, etc.

Answer (*d*).

Some of the monogenic traits are albinism, achondroplasia and neurofibromatosis. Polygenic traits are hereditary and typically exert control over rather common characteristics such as height, skin pigmentation, and intelligence. Genetic control takes place through many gene loci collectively asserting their regulation of the trait.

6. Individuals affected with heritable syndromes involving the face often look more like others with the same disease who are not genetically related than they do their own siblings. Which of the following is an example of this?

(*a*) Down syndrome.

(*b*) Hereditary ectodermal dysplasia.

(*c*) Infantile hypercalcemia syndrome.

(*d*) Stickler syndrome.

(*e*) All of the above.

Answer (*e*).

Individuals affected with the above mentioned syndromes have a striking similarity to each other.

7. The term multifactorial inheritance has been employed to describe traits that do not fit simple mendelian inheritance pattern. A multifactorial inheritance disorder is one that is determined by environmental factors only.

(*a*) Both the statements are true.

(*b*) Both the statements are false.

(*c*) First statement is true and the second is false.

(*d*) First statement is false and the second is true.

Answer (*c*).

A multifactorial inheritance disorder is one that is determined by a combination of genetic and environmental factors. Dental caries, malocclusion and periodontal disease are examples of diseases with multifactorial etiology. Some of the common systemic disorders which are multifactorial in etiology are diabetes, hypertension, etc.

8. While evaluating genetic traits, the first affected individual in a family who brings that family to attention is referred to as the:

(*a*) proband (*b*) propositus

(*c*) index case (*d*) any of the above

Answer (*d*).

The affected individual in a family who first brings that family to the attention of the geneticist is called the proband or propositus. This individual is also known as the index case.

9. The clinical appearance of a given trait for an individual, such as eye colour or height is the individual's genotype. The specific genetic make-up that controls that genotype is the phenotype.

(*a*) Both the statements are true.

(*b*) Both the statements are false.

(*c*) First statement is true and the second is false.

(*d*) First statement is false and the second is true.

Answer (*b*).

The clinical appearance of a given trait for an individual, such as eye colour or height is the individual's phenotype whereas the specific genetic make-up that controls the phenotype is the genotype.

10. A gene that expresses a particular phenotype in a single dose is a recessive gene. If the gene must be present in double dose (homozygous) to express a phenotype it is a dominant gene.

(*a*) Both the statements are true.

(*b*) Both the statements are false.

(*c*) First statement is true and the second is false.

(*d*) First statement is false and the second is true.

Answer (*b*).

A gene that expresses a particular phenotype in a single dose is a dominant gene. If the gene must be present in double dose (homozygous) to express a phenotype it is recessive gene.

11. Which of the following general criteria for making the diagnosis of autosomal dominant inheritance is incorrect?

(*a*) The trait appears in each generation.

(*b*) On an average 100% of the offsprings of affected parents will also be affected.

(*c*) Unaffected parents do not have an affected offspring. There are two important exceptions: a fresh gene mutation in one of the parental gametes and when the trait shows non-penetrance.

(*d*) The occurrence and transmission of the trait are not affected by sex. Males and females are equally likely to have or transmit the trait.

Answer (*b*).

In autosomal dominant inheritance an average of 50% of the offspring of affected parents will be affected.

12. Which of the following criteria about autosomal recessive inheritance is true?

(*a*) The trait typically appears only in siblings, not in parents or other relatives.

(*b*) On an average 1/4th of the siblings of an affected individual will be similarly affected.

(*c*) The rarer the trait the more likely that the parental meeting is consanguineous.

(*d*) Males and females are equally likely to be affected.

(*e*) All of the above.

Answer (*e*).

The answer is self-explanatory.

13. Dentinogenesis imperfecta is inherited as an autosomal dominant trait, has practically 100% penetrance, since all individuals who carry that gene show the phenotype. But Osteogenesis imperfecta shows incomplete penetrance since pedigree studies have demonstrated individuals who carry the gene but do not appear to be affected themselves.

(*a*) Both the statements are true.

(*b*) Both the statements are false.

(*c*) First statement is true and the second is false.

(*d*) First statement is false and the second is true.

Answer (*a*).

The answer is self-explanatory.

14. Cardinal features of Osteogenesis imperfecta is/are:

(*a*) multiple fractures

(*b*) blue sclera

(*c*) dentinogenesis Imperfecta

(*d*) otosclerosis

(*e*) all of the above

Answer (*e*).

All of the above are characteristic featrues of Osteogenesis imperfecta.

15. Monogenic traits have a low recurrence rate. multifactorial traits have a very high recurrence rate.

(*a*) Both the statements are true.

(*b*) Both the statements are false.

(*c*) First statement is true and the second is false.

(*d*) First statement is false and the second is true.

Answer (*b*).

Monogenic traits have a high recurrence rate. Multifactorial traits have a very low recurrence rate.

16. Monozygotic twins result from a single ovum fertilized by a single sperm. Dizygotic twins result from fertilization of two ova by two sperms.

(*a*) Both the statements are true.

(*b*) Both the statements are false.

(*c*) First statement is true and the second is false.

(*d*) First statement is false and the second is true.

Answer (*a*).

The answer is self-explanatory.

17. Which of the following syndromes show periodontal destruction as one of its clinical features?

(*a*) Ehler Danlos syndrome type VIII.

(*b*) Histiocytosis X disease.

(*c*) Papillon-Lefevre syndrome.

(*d*) All of the above.

Answer (*d*).

Genetic conditions that predispose to periodontal disease, such as leucocyte adhesion deficiencies, Chediak-Higashi syndrome, cyclic neutropenia, and papillon Lefevre syndrome have been associated with impaired function of phagocytes or phagocyte adherence to the walls of the blood vessels.

18. In which race (country) is malocclusion virtually non-existent?

(*a*) Japanese. (*b*) Negro.

(*c*) Philipinos. (*d*) Chinese.

Answer (*c*).

Dental anthropologists feel that malocclusion is uncommon in pure racial populations. This could be because of lack of procreation with other populations or a less refined diet often eaten by these typically isolated groups.

19. BRAX – I gene is associated with:

(*a*) dentin formation

(*b*) enamel formation

(*c*) cementum formation

(*d*) alveolar bone formation

Answer (*b*).

The answer is self-explanatory.

20. Proline rich proteins in saliva are associated with:

(*a*) 11th chromosome

(*b*) 12th chromosome

(*c*) 4th chromosome

(*d*) 1st chromosome

Answer (*b*).

Proline rich proteins are associated with the genes located in the 12th chromosome in 12p13.2 region.

Chapter 22

Radiographic Techniques

1. X-rays was discovered by:

(*a*) Roentgen (*b*) Fleming

(*c*) Crooks (*d*) Craig

Answer (*a*).

Roentgen discovered X-rays in 1895.

2. Discovery of X-rays was made in:

(*a*) 1895 (*b*) 1905

(*c*) 1960 (*d*) 1885

Answer (*a*).

Refer to the explanation of Q. No. 1.

3. Dental radiography began:

(*a*) 10 weeks after discovery of X-rays

(*b*) 6 months after discovery of X-rays

(*c*) 6 weeks after discovery of X-rays

(*d*) 6 days after discovery of X-rays

Answer (*c*).

Six weeks after Roentgen's announcement of discovery of X-rays, a dentist attempted to record shadows of oral structures on a film. Although they were crude images dental radiography had begun.

4. The selection of appropriate radiographs for the pediatric patient depends on:

(*a*) the age of the child

(*b*) size of the oral cavity

(*c*) level of patient co-operation

(*d*) all of the above

Answer (*d*).

The selection of appropriate radiographs for the pediatric patient depends on all of the above mentioned factors.

5. X-rays cause biologic damage by:

(*a*) immediate cell death

(*b*) enhancing autolysis or apoptosis

(*c*) imparting its energy and causing injury to the tissues through which it traverses

(*d*) stimulating killer T cells

Answer (*c*).

One characteristic feature of X-rays is its ability to impart some of its energy to the matter it traverses. If the matter is living tissue then biologic injury may occur.

6. Biologic damage caused by X-rays can be:

(*a*) carcinogenesis (*b*) mutagenesis

(*c*) teratogenesis (*d*) any of the above

Answer (*d*).

Carcinogenesis and malformations are the response of somatic tissues and in most instances are believed to have a threshold (that is a certain amount of radiation is necessary for the response to be seen). Mutation may occur as a response of genetic tissue to X-radiation and is believed to have no threshold. In general, younger tissues and organs are more sensitive to radiation (with the sensitivity decreasing from the period before birth until maturity).

7. Natural background radiation normally is:

(*a*) 102–120 mrem/year

(*b*) 202–220 mrem/year

(*c*) 92 mrem/year

(*d*) 250–300 mrem/year

Answer (*a*).

The answer is self-explanatory. In milli sievert it is 1.02 to 1.20.

8. Radiation induced damage most often will result in cancer of the following organs except:

(*a*) skin (*b*) breast

(*c*) thyroid (*d*) gonads

Answer (*d*).

In gonads radiation causes mutations, infertility and fetal malformations whereas in skin, breasts and thyroid it causes cancer.

9. The fastest film available for dental radiography is:

(*a*) A (*b*) B

(*c*) E (*d*) D

Answer (*c*).

Faster film speeds have contributed most significantly to the reduction in radiation to the patient. Film speeds of D and E are currently available for dental radiography.

10. All of the following decrease the radiation exposure to the patient except:

(*a*) using a lead apron and a thyroid collar

(*b*) using high kilovolt peak

(*c*) using slow speed film

(*d*) using filters and diaphragms

Answer (*c*).

Use of slow speed film increases the exposure time thereby increasing the exposure of the patient to the radiation. The lead apron protects the gonads and the chest from the primary beam and scatter radiation whereas the collar shields the thyroid.

11. A 4-year-old child with no apparent abnormalities and open contacts should undergo:

(*a*) 4 film survey

(*b*) 8 film survey

(*c*) no radiographic examination

(*d*) 12 film survey

Answer (*c*).

When there are open proximal contacts one need not undergo radiographic examination.

12. Four film series consists of all except:

(*a*) anterior occlusal maxillary

(*b*) anterior occlusal mandibular

(*c*) bitewings

(*d*) OPG

Answer (*d*).

Refer to the explanation below:

Four film survey	– Maxillary anterior occlusal Mandibular anterior occlusal Two posterior bitewings
Eight film survey	– Maxillary/Mandibular anterior occlusal (or periapicals) Right, left, maxillary posterior occlusal (or periapicals) Right, left, mandibular primary molar periapicals Two posterior bitewings
Twelve film survey	– Four primary molar/premolar periapicals Four canine periapicals Two incisor periapicals Two posterior bitewings
Sixteen film survey	– 12-film survey + Four permanent molar periapicals.

13. All of the following are correct regarding 12-film survey except:

(*a*) four primary molars/premolar periapicals

(*b*) four canine periapicals

(*c*) two incisor periapicals

(*d*) two molar periapicals

Answer (*d*).

Refer to the explanation of Q. No. 12.

14. The size of the film commonly used for bitewing radiography is:

(*a*) 0 and 4 (*b*) 0 and 2

(*c*) 2 and 4 (*d*) 1 and 2

Answer (*b*).

The answer is self-explanatory.

15. During bitewing radiography the ala-tragus line is:

(*a*) parallel to the floor

(*b*) perpendicular to the floor

(*c*) the position of the ala-tragus line is not significant

(*d*) parallel to the occlusal plane

Answer (*a*).

While taking a bitewing radiograph the head is positioned so that the mid-sagittal plane is perpendicular and the ala-tragus line is parallel to the floor.

16. Which of the corners of the film is to be folded while taking a bitewing radiograph?

(*a*) Anterosuperior and posteroinferior.

(*b*) Posterosuperior and anteroinferior.

(*c*) Posterosuperior and posteroinferior.

(*d*) Anteroinferior and posterosuperior.

Answer (*b*).

Anteroinferior corner is bent to prevent damage to the lingual frenum and posterosuperior corner is bent to prevent gagging.

17. The vertical angulation for bitewing radiography is:

(*a*) +8 (*b*) +12

(*c*) –8 (*d*) –12

Answer (*a*).

The vertical angulation for bitewing radiography is +8 to +10 degrees.

18. Bisecting angle and paralleling techniques are used to take:

(*a*) periapical radiographs

(*b*) bitewing radiographs

(*c*) occlusal radiographs

(*d*) mandibular occlusal view

Answer (*a*).

The answer is self-explanatory.

19. In paralleling technique the film is placed (for maxillary radiography):

(*a*) close to the object

(*b*) far from the object

(*c*) object-film distance is not a criteria

(*d*) none of the above

Answer (*b*).

The paralleling technique requires the object and film to be parallel in all dimensions. To achieve this, the film packet is placed farther away from the object, particularly in the maxilla.

20. All of the following are true regarding the bisecting angle technique except:

(*a*) it is based on rule of isometry

(*b*) the central X-ray is directed perpendicular to the bisector (*c*) it is used to take periapical radiographs

(*d*) the accuracy is better than that of the paralleling technique

Answer (*d*).

The rule of isometry states that two triangles are equal if they have two equal angles and a common side. Radiographs taken by paralleling technique have better contrast and accuracy than bisecting angle technique.

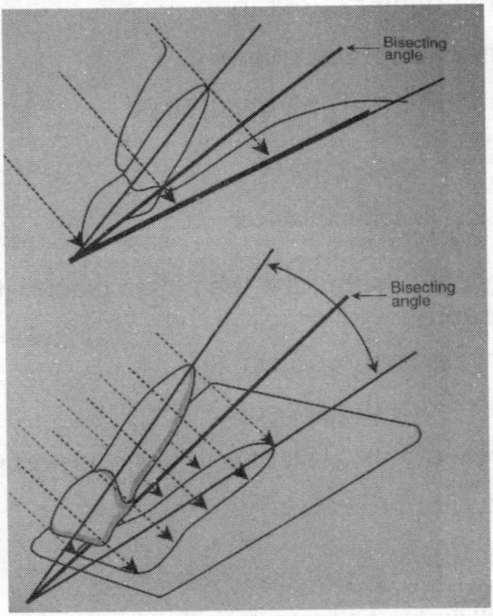

Fig. 22.1 Rule of isometry—Bisecting angle technique.

21. Orthopantamography:

(*a*) uses a mechanism by which the X-ray film and the source move in opposite directions

(*b*) needs complete immobility for approximately 5–22 seconds (*c*) is a supplement for intraoral periapical radiographic series

(*d*) all of the above

Answer (*d*).

The answer is self-explanatory.

22. The normal range of Kvp for intraoral radiography is:

(*a*) 20–40 Kvp (*b*) 80–120 Kvp

(*c*) 60–90 Kvp (*d*) more than 120 Kvp

Answer (*b*).

The use of higher kilovolt peak techniques reduces patient exposure to radiation and lowers the contrast thus increasing the number of shades of gray on the film.

23. Bitewing radiographs of a 5-year-old child show interproximal caries just short of DE junction. The dentist should recommend:

(*a*) restoration of the tooth as soon as possible

(*b*) prophylaxis and topical fluoride application

(*c*) disking of the affected areas

(*d*) three month recall for re-evaluation

Answer (*a*).

Interproximal caries in the primary molars involve the pulp faster. Hence, restoration as soon as it is detected is the treatment of choice.

24. When no new decay is formed the frequency of repeated bitewing radiographs recommended in permanent dentition is:

(*a*) once in every 18–24 months

(*b*) once in every 12–18 months

(*c*) once in 48 months

(*d*) once a year

Answer (*a*).

If no evidence of caries is found, then X-rays may be taken every 12–18 months if primary teeth are in contact or every 18–24 months if permanent teeth are in contact.

25. According to buccal object rule, the object that is present in the buccal side:

(*a*) moves in the same direction

(*b*) moves in the opposite direction

(*c*) remains static

(*d*) none of the above

Answer (*b*).

The object localization technique uses the SLOB rule. It says that if the object is present on the buccal side it moves in the opposite direction and if it is in the lingual side it moves in the Same direction.

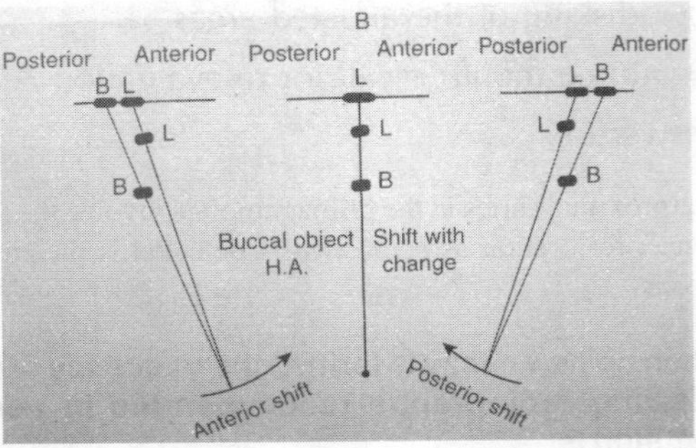

Fig. 22.2 SLOB rule.

26. For all maxillary films, the ala-tragus line is:

(*a*) parallel to the floor

(*b*) perpendicular to the floor

(*c*) parallel to the occlusal plane

(*d*) none of the above

Answer (*a*).

The answer is self-explanatory. Refer to the explanation of Q. No. 15.

27. When a panoramic radiograph is possible the ideal survey for primary dentition with closed contacts is:

(*a*) OPG only

(*b*) OPG and a pair of bitewings

(*c*) OPG and a pair of bitewings and 2 periapicals

(*d*) OPG and two occlusal view

Answer (*c*).

A pair of bitewings evaluates the proximal areas while the two anterior periapicals assess the anterior teeth and the OPG gives the overall status of the dental development.

28. To utilize the buccal object rule for object localization one has to take:

(*a*) 1 radiograph (*b*) 2 radiographs

(*c*) 3 radiographs (*d*) 4 radiographs

Answer (*b*).

Two radiographs have to be taken to utilize the SLOB rule. The first film is taken as a routine radiograph. The second film is placed in the same position. The head position and the vertical angle remains the same but the horizontal angle is shifted either anteriorly or posteriorly.

29. Panoramic radiographs are least useful in demonstrating:

(*a*) supernumerary tooth

(*b*) incipient carious lesion

(*c*) congenitally missing tooth

(*d*) axial inclinations of teeth

Answer (*b*).

Good bitewing radiographs usually detect incipient caries. In OPG the proximal surfaces are usually overlapped which makes it a poor indicator of proximal caries.

Chapter 23

Tumours and Cysts of Oral Cavity in Children

1. Oral warts are caused by:

(*a*) human papilloma virus

(*b*) pox virus

(*c*) hepatitis B virus

(*d*) rota virus

Answer (*a*).

Oral verruca vulgaris or oral warts are exophytic papillomatous lesions indistinguishable clinically from oral squamous cell papillomas. They are caused by Human Papilloma Virus. This virus could be an etiological agent in cervical cancer of uterus.

2. The most common benign soft-tissue tumour found in the oral cavity is:

(*a*) verrruca vulgaris

(*b*) squamous papilloma

(*c*) fibroma

(*d*) pyogenic granuloma

Answer (*c*).

Fibroma is a dome shaped lesion with a sessile base and a smooth surface that usually has the colour of the surrounding mucosa.

3. Which of the following are true about oral verruca vulgaris or oral warts?

(*a*) They are exophytic papillomatous lesions indistinguishable clinically from oral squamous cell neoplasms.

(*b*) They are caused by human papilloma virus.

(*c*) They can spread to the oral cavity in children through autoinoculation by finger or thumb sucking.

(*d*) Complete surgical excision including the base is the treatment of choice.

(*e*) All of the above.

Answer (*e*).

The answer is self-explanatory.

4. Which of the following are true about pyogenic granuloma?

(*a*) Soft tissue tumour arises from fibrous connective tissue or mucous membranes.

(*b*) Surface may have a smooth, lobulated or occasionally warty appearance that is erythematous and often ulcerated.

(*c*) Because of the pronounced vascularity, these lesions often bleed easily when probed.

(*d*) Commonly occurring sites are maxillary anterior labial gingiva, lips,tongue,buccal mucosa, palate, mucolabial or mucobuccal fold.

(*e*) All of the above.

Answer (*e*).

The answer is self-explanatory.

5. Ranula is the clinical term for a mucocele occurring on the floor of the mouth after trauma to components of the submandibular glands. Two varieties of ranula exist: cystic (mucous retention cyst) and pseudocystic (mucous retention phenomenon or mucocele).

(*a*) Both the statements are false.

(*b*) Both the statements are true.

(*c*) First statement is true and the second is false.

(*d*) First statement is false and the second is true.

Answer (*d*).

Ranula is the clinical term for a mucocele occurring on the floor of the mouth after trauma to components of the sublingual glands.

6. In the cystic type of mucocele, there is partial obstruction of the distal end of a sublingual gland duct that results in a small epithelial lined cyst usually less than 1 cm in diameter. The most common variety of ranula (which is pseudocystic) however forms as a result of extravasation of mucous into the fibrous connective tissue after a tear in the sublingual gland duct.

(*a*) Both the statements are false.

(*b*) Both the statements are true.

(*c*) First statement is true and the second is false.

(*d*) First statement is false and the second is true.

Answer (*b*).

The answer is self-explanatory.

7. Mucoceles are rarely seen in:

(*a*) upper lip (*b*) lower lip

(*c*) buccal mucosa (*d*) floor of the mouth

Answer (*a*).

Mucoceles are noted to occur most commonly on the lower lip, with the floor of the mouth and buccal mucosa being the next most frequent sites of involvement. They are rarely seen on the upper lip, retromolar pad or palate.

8. The commonest site of occurrence of congenital epulis of newborn is:

(*a*) mandibular anterior alveolar ridge

(*b*) maxillary anterior alveolar ridge

(*c*) maxillary posterior alveolar ridge

(*d*) mandibular posterior alveolar ridge

Answer (*b*).

Congenital epulis of newborn is a rare lesion of uncertain histogenesis that occurs exclusively in newborn infants chiefly on the maxillary anterior alveolar ridge and less commonly on the mandibular anterior alveolar ridge. Usually they are solitary lesions but they may be multiple also, often affecting both the maxilla and mandible. At birth it presents as pink, smooth to lobulated, pedunculated mass that may vary in size from a few millimeters to greater than 7 cm in diameter. More than 90% of cases occur in females.

9. Neurofibroma is a benign neural neoplasm of Schwann cell origin for which several clinical forms are recognized. It is an autosomal recessive inherited disease.

(*a*) Both the statements are false.

(*b*) Both the statements are true.

(*c*) First statement is true and the second is false.

(*d*) First statement is false and the second is true.

Answer (*c*).

Neurofibroma is inherited as an autosomal dominant disease.

10. Which of the following conditions exist in neurofibromatosis?

(*a*) Café-au-lait spots.

(*b*) Lisch nodules.

(*c*) Pigmented iris hamartomas.

(*d*) All of the above.

Answer (*d*).

Café – Coffee, Lait – Milk. (When coffee is mixed with milk the resulting colour is brown.) Hence it is called Café-au-lait spots. They are light brown macules with smooth borders and often located over nerve trunks. This is seen in type I neurofibromatosis (von Recklinghausen's disease). Lisch nodules – pigmented hamartomas in the iris present in more than 94% of patients who are 6 years old or older. They do not produce any symptoms but are helpful in establishing the diagnosis.

11. The most frequent intra oral location for neurofibromatosis is palate or floor of the mouth. Occasionally intraosseous lesion occurs in the posterior part of the mandible.

(*a*) Both the statements are false.

(*b*) Both the statements are true.

(*c*) First statement is true and the second is false.

(*d*) First statement is false and the second is true.

Answer (*d*).

The most frequent intra oral location for neurofibromatosis is tongue or buccal mucosa.

12. Lymphangiomas are thought to arise as benign hamartomatous proliferations of sequestrated lymphatic rests. They form along tissue planes or penetrating adjacent tissue; they become canalized and in the congenital absence of venous drainage accumulate fluid.

(*a*) Both the statements are false.

(*b*) Both the statements are true.

(*c*) First statement is true and the second is false.

(*d*) First statement is false and the second is true.

Answer (*b*).

The answer is self-explanatory. Lymphangiomas are classified into three types: Capillary lymphangiomas, cavernous lymphangiomas and cystic hygroma.

13. Hemangioma is a benign vasoformative tumor that frequently occurs in the head and neck in children. Most hemangiomas develop when the child is 5–8 years of age.

(*a*) Both the statements are false.

(*b*) Both the statements are true.

(*c*) First statement is true and the second is false.

(*d*) First statement is false and the second is true.

Answer (*c*).

Most hemangiomas are either present at birth or develop within the first year of life.

14. Hemangiomas in the oral soft tissues commonly affect palate and floor of the mouth. Their histologic classification is based on the type of the blood vessels involved.

(*a*) Both the statements are false.

(*b*) Both the statements are true.

(*c*) First statement is true and the second is false.

(*d*) First statement is false and the second is true.

Answer (*a*).

Hemangiomas in the oral soft tissues commonly affect tongue, lips and buccal mucosa. Their histologic classification is based on the size of the vascular spaces. They are classified as capillary, cavernous, central and cellular hemangiomas.

15. The fibro-osseous lesions of the jaws include a diverse group of lesions sharing a common denominator, the replacement of normal bone architecture by a benign fibro cellular stroma. Because of their histomorphology, diagnosis is made on the basis of distinguishing clinical and radiographic features.

(*a*) Both the statements are false.

(*b*) Both the statements are true.

(*c*) First statement is true and the second is false.

(*d*) First statement is false and the second is true.

Answer (*b*).

The answer is self-explanatory. Fibrous dysplasia and the ossifying fibroma are the common fibroosseous lesions in children.

16. All of the following statements are true regarding fibrous dysplasia except:

(*a*) it is a neoplastic developmental lesion of the bone

(*b*) two forms exist: rare polyostotic form and common monoostotic form

(*c*) maxillary involvement is a more serious form of disease

(*d*) radiographically they show a ground glass appearance

Answer (*a*).

Fibrous dysplasia is a non-neoplastic lesion of the bone. The other three statements are true regarding fibrous dysplasia.

17. Which of the following is/are true regarding monosostotic fibrous dysplasia?

(*a*) Slow growing and painless.

(*b*) Progressive enlargement of bone whose growth pattern stabilizes with time frequently after the onset of puberty.

(*c*) The margins are ill defined and blend into normal bone necessitating conservative therapy.

(*d*) All of the above.

Answer (*d*).

The answer is self-explanatory. Surgery in the form of osseous recontouring should be considered only in those cases where there is functional or significant cosmetic deformity and usually after stabilization of the disease process.

18. Which of the following fibro-osseous lesion is of periodontal ligament origin?

(*a*) Fibrous dysplasia.

(*b*) Ossifying fibroma.

(*c*) Central giant cell granuloma.

(*d*) Peripheral giant cell granuloma.

Answer (*b*).

The ossifying fibroma is a benign fibro-osseous neoplasm of periodontal ligament origin included in the broad category of benign fibro-osseous lesions of the jaws. It is characterized histologically by benign fibro cellular stroma, with the formation of variable amounts of woven bone, lamellar bone, and spherical to annular to amorphous cementum like calcifications. When the predominant calcified component is bone it is known as ossifying fibroma. On the other hand if cementum or cementum like calcifications predominate it is known as cementifying fibroma.

19. Which of the following is true regarding central giant cell granuloma?

(*a*) 50% of the patients are less than 16 years of age.

(*b*) Occurs more often in females than males.

(*c*) Mandible is involved more than maxilla.

(*d*) All of the above.

Answer (*d*).

The answer is self-explanatory. Majority of the lesions occur in the anterior portion of the maxilla (anterior to 1st permanent molar).

20. The cyst formed by cystic degeneration of enamel organ is:

(*a*) dentigerous cyst
(*b*) primordial cyst
(*c*) odontogenic keratocyst
(*d*) eruption cyst

Answer (*b*).

Cyst formed by the cystic degeneration of the enamel organ before the formation of enamel or dentin is known as primordial cyst.

21. A patient aged 12 years reports with a swelling in the left mandibular premolar region. Radio graphically there is a well-circumscribed, unilocular radiolucent lesion where the first premolar failed to develop and there was no history of extraction before. The probable diagnosis is:

(*a*) dentigerous cyst
(*b*) primordial cyst
(*c*) odontogenic keratocyst
(*d*) eruption cyst

Answer (*b*).

Refer to the explanation of Q. No. 20.

22. The cyst which is associated with erupting primary and permanent tooth in its soft tissue phase after erupting through bone is:

(*a*) dentigerous cyst
(*b*) primordial cyst
(*c*) odontogenic keratocyst
(*d*) eruption cyst

Answer (*d*).

Eruption cyst is usually a translucent, smooth, painless swelling over the erupting tooth. If bleeding occurs into the cystic space, it may appear blue to blue-black and it is then called an eruption hematoma.

23. The cyst which is associated with the crown of an impacted, embedded or unerupted tooth is:

(*a*) dentigerous cyst

(*b*) primordial cyst

(*c*) odontogenic keratocyst

(*d*) eruption cyst

Answer (*a*).

Dentigerous cysts are usually large, destructive and expansile lesions of bone. The radiographic appearance may be unilocular or multilocular.

24. All of the following are true about odontogenic keratocyst except:

(*a*) it has a high rate of recurrence

(*b*) peak incidence is in second and third decades of life

(*c*) maxilla is involved twice as frequently as the mandible

(*d*) histologically it has a thin uniform lining epithelium with palisading of basal layer of cells and a corrugated surface

Answer (*c*).

Odontogenic keratocyst involves mandible twice as frequently as the maxilla.

25. Ameloblastoma found in children is usually the polycystic variety.The most common histopathologic picture found in Ameloblastoma in children is Plexiform variety.

(*a*) Both the statements are false.

(*b*) Both the statements are true.

(*c*) First statement is true and the second is false.

(*d*) First statement is false and the second is true.

Answer (*d*).

Ameloblastoma found in children is usually the unicystic variety.

26. The most common site for Ameloblastoma in children is:

(*a*) mandibular anterior region

(*b*) mandibular molar ramus area

(*c*) maxillary antrum

(*d*) maxillary posterior region

Answer (*b*).

The answer is self-explanatory.

27. All of the following are true about adenomatoid odontogenic tumour except:

(*a*) otherwise known as adenoameloblastoma

(*b*) classified as intraosseous (follicular and extrafollicular) and extraosseous variants

(*c*) occurs most commonly in the second decade of life

(*d*) occurs most commonly in the mandibular incisor and canine region

Answer (*d*).

Adenomatoid odontogenic tumour occurs nearly twice as frequently in the maxilla as in the mandible, with a noticeable predilection for occurrence in the canine and incisor regions.

28. The most common and least severe form of Histiocytosis X, when the disease is confined to bone is known as:

(*a*) Hand-Schuller-Christian disease

(*b*) Eosinophilic granuloma

(*c*) Letterer-Siwe disease

(*d*) histiocytosis Y

Answer (*b*).

Eosinophilic granuloma is the most common and least severe form of LCH, if that form of the disease is confined to bone. Langerhans cell histiocytosis is the current term replacing the term Histiocytosis X introduced by Lichtenstein in 1953 as a unifying term for several previous eponyms including Letterer-Siwe disease, Hand-Schuller-Christian disease and Eosinophilic granuloma.

29. All of the following are true regarding Eosinophilic granuloma except:

(*a*) characterized by single or multiple well-defined radiolucent bony lesions and occasionally accompanied by pain and swelling

(*b*) older children and young adults are most commonly affected

(*c*) mandible, skull, femur, humerus, ribs and pelvis are frequently involved

(*d*) skin and visceral involvement is common

Answer (*d*).

Skin and visceral involvement are absent (similar to Hand-Schuller-Christian disease and Letterer-Siwe disease).

30. Which of the following is the chronic disseminated form of Histiocytosis X?

(*a*) Hand-Schuller-Christian disease

(*b*) Eosinophilic granuloma

(*c*) Letterer-Siwe disease

(*d*) Histiocytosis Y

Answer (*a*).

The term Hand-Schuller-Christian disease is used to describe the chronic, disseminated form of LCH and is characterized by the development of multifocal eosinophilic granulomas of bone, lymphadenopathy and visceral involvement especially hepatosplenomegaly.

31. The classical triad of multiple punched out radiolucent lesions of membranous bones, exophthalmos, and diabetes insipidus is characteristic of:

(*a*) Hand-Schuller-Christian disease

(*b*) eosinophilic granuloma

(*c*) letterer-Siwe disease

(*d*) histiocytosis Y

Answer (*a*).

The answer is self-explanatory.

32. Which of the following is characterized initially by a development of a scaly erythematous skin rash?

(*a*) Hand-Schuller-Christian disease

(*b*) Eosinophilic granuloma

(*c*) Letterer-Siwe disease

(*d*) Histiocytosis Y

Answer (*c*).

This scaly rash is initially prominent on the trunk but progressing to involve the scalp and extremities. This is accompanied by a persistent low-grade fever, anemia, thrombocytopenia, hepatosplenomegaly and lymphadenopathy.

33. Which of the following is true regarding Ewing's sarcoma?

(*a*) It usually affects the skull, mandible and the maxilla in the head and neck region.

(*b*) Localized pain and swelling are the most frequent complaints at the time of presentation.

(*c*) Soft tissue overlying the swelling may be erythematous and warm to touch suggestive of an inflammatory process than a neoplasm.

(*d*) Any of the above.

Answer (*d*).

The answer is self-explanatory. Following osteosarcoma,the Ewing's family of tumors is the second most common primary malignancy of bone in children and adolescence.

34. Sun ray appearance in the radiograph is characteristic of:

(*a*) osteogenic sarcoma

(*b*) ewing's sarcoma

(*c*) hand-Schuller-Christain disease

(*d*) rhabdomyosarcoma

Answer (*a*).

A frequently described radiographic feature of Osteogenic sarcoma is a sun-ray appearance, with delicate, hairlike trabeculae radiating in a sunburst fashion away from the peripheral surface of the lesion.

35. All of the following are true regarding Rhabdomyosarcoma except:

(*a*) a benign neoplasm of skeletal muscle origin

(*b*) most common soft tissue sarcoma in children

(*c*) 2–6 years and adolescence are the commonly affected age group

(*d*) Primary site of involvement in children is the head and neck region

Answer (*a*).

Rhabdomyosarcoma is a malignant neoplasm of skeletal muscle origin.

36. Presence of Reed-Sternberg cells is characteristic of:

(*a*) non-Hodgkin's lymphoma

(*b*) Hodgkin's lymphoma

(*c*) Burkitt's Lymphoma

(*d*) Rhabdomyosarcoma

Answer (*b*)

Hodgkin's disease is a malignant neoplasm of lymphoreticular origin distinguished from Non-Hodgkins lymphoma by diverse but distinctive morphologic features with one common denominator, the presence of Reed-Sternberg cells which are widely accepted as the neoplastic cells in this disease.

Chapter 24

Developmental Disturbances of Teeth

1. The most common microorganism associated with a periapical infection, which results in an alveolar abscess, is:

(*a*) Staphylococcus

(*b*) Streptococcus viridans

(*c*) Pneumococci

(*d*) Staphylococcus salivarius

Answer (*b*).

The Streptococcus viridans group of microorganisms produce significant amounts of hyaluronidase and fibrinolysins which act to break down or dissolve hyaluronic acid and fibrin.

2. While making an access opening in an abscessed tooth the discomfort can be lessened if the tooth is stabilized by the dentist's finger. A splint of impression compound can also stabilize the tooth:

(*a*) both the statements are false

(*b*) both the statements are true

(*c*) first statement is true and the second is false

(*d*) first statement is false and the second is true

Answer (*b*).

When the tooth is stabilized, the pressure exerted in the apical direction by the hand piece and the bur is reduced. This reduces the pain and discomfort.

3. In Ludwig's angina, all of the following spaces are involved except:

(*a*) submental space (*b*) submandibular space

(*c*) sublingual space (*d*) pterygoid space

Answer (*d*).

Cellulitis from an infected mandibular tooth can spread to the floor of the mouth along fascial planes, nerves and vessels. If the infection involves the submandibular, sublingual and submental spaces, it is called Ludwig's angina. In this condition the tongue and floor of the mouth is elevated to the extent that the patient's airway gets obstructed and swallowing becomes impossible.

4. Which of the following is the spreading factor that causes the infection to spread into the tissue spaces in Ludwig's angina?

(*a*) Collagenase.

(*b*) Hyaluronic acid.

(*c*) Hyaluronidase.

(*d*) Polysachharidase.

Answer (*c*).

Hyaluronidase breaks down the intercellular cementing substance (hyaluronic acid). Similarly fibrinolysin breaks down the fibrin. This leads to a rapid spread of the infection.

5. Continued budding of the primary or permanent tooth germ as a result of an abnormal proliferation of cells of the tooth germ results in:

(*a*) dentigerous cyst

(*b*) odontoma

(*c*) anodontia

(*d*) odontogenic keratocyst

Answer (*b*).

The question explains the etiology of odontoma.

6. Treatment for odontoma is usually:

(*a*) observation (*b*) surgical excision

(*c*) allowing it to erupt (*d*) orthodontic extrusion

Answer (*b*).

Odontomas are usually removed surgically before they interfere with the eruption of adjacent teeth.

7. All of the following are true about fusion except:

(*a*) they follow a familial tendency

(*b*) union of two independently developing primary or permanent teeth

(*c*) when there is fusion in primary teeth, congenital absence of the corresponding permanent teeth is never seen

(*d*) fused teeth have separate pulp chambers and separate pulp canals

Answer (*c*).

A frequent finding in fusion of primary teeth is the congenital absence of one of the corresponding permanent teeth.

8. All of the following about Gemination are true except:

(*a*) it represents an attempted division of a single tooth germ by invagination

(*b*) it does not follow a hereditary pattern

(*c*) it appears clinically as a bifid crown on a single root

(*d*) it is seen in both primary and permanent teeth

Answer (*b*).

Gemination follows a hereditary pattern of occurrence, seen in both primary and permanent teeth but more frequently in primary teeth.

9. Dens in Dente is most often seen in:

(*a*) permanent maxillary central incisors

(*b*) permanent maxillary lateral incisors

(*c*) primary maxillary lateral incisors

(*d*) primary mandibular lateral incisors

Answer (*b*).

This condition should be suspected whenever deep lingual pits are observed in maxillary permanent lateral incisors.

10. Which of the following regarding dens in dente is true?

(*a*) this condition should be suspected whenever deep lingual pits are observed in maxillary permanent lateral incisors

(*b*) this condition can occur in primary and permanent teeth (*c*) prophylactic application of a sealant or restoration is indicated

(*d*) if the condition is detected before the complete eruption of the tooth, the removal of gingival tissue to facilitate cavity preparation and restoration may be indicated

(*e*) all of the above

Answer (*e*).

The answer is self-explanatory.

11. Variations in the time of eruption of primary teeth and in the time of exfoliation are frequently observed in pediatric patients. How much of variation in time in exfoliation of primary teeth is considered normal?

(*a*) 6 months. (*b*) 18 months.

(*c*) 36 months. (*d*) 48 months.

Answer (*b*).

A variation of 18 months in the exfoliation time of primary teeth may be considered normal. Exfoliation of teeth in the absence of trauma in children younger than 5 years of age merits special attention because it can be related to pathologic conditions of local and systemic region.

12. All of the following are true regarding Cherubism except:

(*a*) it is otherwise known as familial fibrous dysplasia

(*b*) numerous sharp,well defined multilocular areas of bone destruction and thinning of cortical plate are usually evident in radiograph (*c*) it is characterized by delayed exfoliation of primary teeth

(*d*) it has an autosomal dominant pattern of inheritance

Answer (*c*).

In Cherubism, teeth are frequently exfoliated prematurely as a result of loss of support or root resorption or in permanent teeth as a result of interference with the development of roots. Spontaneous loss of teeth may occur or the child may pick the teeth out of the soft tissue.

13. Which of the following about Acrodynia is true?

(*a*) Exposure of young children to minute amounts of mercury is responsible for this condition.

(*b*) Otherwise known as Pink disease.

(*c*) Ointments and medicaments are the usual sources of mercury and dental amalgam restorations do not cause this condition.

(*d*) Clinical features include fever, anorexia, desquamation of soles and palms, sweating, tachycardia, gastrointestinal disturbance, hypotonia, oral ulcerations, excessive salivation and early exfoliation of primary teeth.

(*e*) All of the above.

Answer (*e*).

The answer is self-explanatory.

14. Micrognathia can be a result of:

(*a*) intrauterine injury and deficient nutrition

(*b*) birth injury

(*c*) infections of temporo-mandibular joint

(*d*) all of the above

Answer (*d*).

Forceps delivery can interfere with the growth of the condyle thereby resulting in micrognathia. Similarly intrauterine injury, deficient nutrition and infections of TMJ can also affect the growth of the condyle resulting in smaller jaws.

15. Which of the following regarding Vitamin D resistant Rickets is true?

(*a*) Also known as familial hypophosphatemia.

(*b*) Inherited usually as an X-linked dominant trait.

(*c*) Absent or abnormal lamina dura is seen in radiographs.

(*d*) Dental manifestations include apical radiolucencies, abscesses and fistulas associated with pulp exposures in primary and permanent teeth.

(*e*) All of the above.

Answer (*e*).

The answer is self-explanatory.

16. All of the following conditions are associated with early exfoliation of teeth except:

(*a*) acrodynia (*b*) Progeria

(*c*) Juvenile diabetes (*d*) Hypopituitarism

Answer (*d*).

Premature exfoliation of teeth is seen in Acrodynia, Progeria and Juvenile diabetes. But in Hypopituitarism there is delayed exfoliation of teeth.

17. All of the following conditions are associated with early exfoliation of teeth except:

(*a*) cherubism

(*b*) hypophosphatasia

(*c*) histiocytosis X

(*d*) hypothyroidism

Answer (*d*).

Premature exfoliation of teeth is seen in Cherubism, Hypophosphatasia and histiocytosis X. But in hypothyroidism there is delayed exfoliation of teeth. Refer to the explanation of Q. No. 16.

18. Local or systemic factors that interfere with the normal matrix formation cause enamel hypocalcification. Factors that interfere with calcification and maturation produces enamel hypoplasia:

(*a*) both the statements are false

(*b*) both the statements are true

(*c*) first statement is true and the second is false

(*d*) first statement is false and the second is true

Answer (*a*).

Interference during matrix formation results in hypoplasia and interference with calcification results in hypocalcification.

19. Which of the following statements regarding primary enamel hypoplasia is/are true?

(*a*) Hypoplasia of primary enamel that forms before birth is rare.

(*b*) It is common in prematurely born, very low birth weight children.

(*c*) If ameloblastic activity is disrupted for a long time, gross areas of irregular enamel occur; if disrupted for a short period of time, it manifests as a thin line or a pit.

(*d*) All of the above.

Answer (*d*).

The answer is self-explanatory.

20. Which of the following is true regarding lead poisoning?

(*a*) The foetus of a lead poisoned mother can be affected because lead readily crosses the placenta during pregnancy.

(*b*) Pica is a common sign of plumbism in children.

(*c*) It can result in pitting hypoplasia.

(*d*) All of the above.

Answer (*d*).

The answer is self-explanatory. Tasting or mouthing of strange objects is normal in children upto age of 2 years. Persistence of this habit beyond the age of two years is termed Pica and it may be a manifestation of parental neglect or lack of affection. The child may develop habit of eating non-edible substances such as sand, clay, paint and wall plaster. These children are prone to lead poisoning and often complain of chronic abdominal pain and pallor.

21. All of the following can result in enamel hypoplasia except:

(*a*) Vit C, D deficiency

(*b*) brain injury and neurologic defects

(*c*) nephrotic syndrome

(*d*) Vit K deficiency

Answer (*d*).

Vitamin K does not have any role in epithelial differentiation or calcification of teeth.

22. All of the following are true regarding Turner's hypoplasia except:

(*a*) it is usually due to local infection

(*b*) it manifests as hypoplastic or hypocalcified areas on the crown of permanent teeth

(*c*) it can be seen in primary teeth also

(*d*) inflammatory processes of primary teeth extend toward the buds of the permanent teeth and affect them during the prefunctional stage of eruption

(*e*) it can be seen in second mandibular premolar.

Answer (*c*).

Turner's hypoplasia occurs usually because of trauma to primary teeth or infection of primary teeth affecting the permanent tooth germ. Hence, it cannot be seen in the primary teeth.

23. Which of the following can be a method of managing enamel hypoplasia?

(*a*) Topical fluoride application.

(*b*) Restoration with glassionomers.

(*c*) Enamel color modification by controlled hydrochloric acid-pumice abrasion.

(*d*) Enamel microabrasion.

(*e*) Any of the above.

Answer (*e*).

Topical fluoride application and glass ionomers are the commonly used strategies. Enamel microabrasion (Croll) is a technique in which a specially prepared abrasive compound (Prema) is applied to the discolored enamel areas, similarly to prophylaxis paste, using a synthetic rubber applicator in a 10:1 gear-reduction handpiece. Frequent water rinsings and reevaluation of the tooth for color correction are required. In the hydrochloric acid technique, slurry of fine pumice and 18% HCl is applied under pressure and abrasion with a wooden stick. The slurry is rinsed away after each 5-second application until the desired color change has occurred.

24. Which of the following is not inherited as an autosomal dominant trait?

(*a*) Dentinogenesis imperfecta.

(*b*) Cherubism.

(*c*) Vit D resistant Rickets (familial hypophosphatemia).

(*d*) Hemophilia.

Answer (*c*).

Vit D resistant rickets is inherited as an X-linked dominant trait.

25. Dentinogenesis imperfecta without Osteogenesis imperfecta is otherwise called:

(*a*) Type I Dentinogenesis imperfecta

(*b*) Type II Dentinogenesis imperfecta

(*c*) Hereditary opalascent dentin

(*d*) both (*b*) and (*c*)

Answer (*d*).

Type I dentinogenesis imperfecta is associated with osteogenesis imperfecta.

Type III dentinogenesis imperfecta is otherwise called Brandywine type.

26. Which of the following is true regarding Dentinogenesis imperfecta?

(*a*) They affect both primary and permanent teeth.

(*b*) The pulp chamber is small or entirely absent and the pulp canals are small and ribbon like.

(*c*) Stainless steel crowns may be considered a means of preventing gross abrasion.

(*d*) Multiple root fractures are present particularly in older patients.

(*e*) All of the above.

Answer (*e*).

All of the above-mentioned statements are true regarding Dentinogenesis imperfecta.

27. All of the following are true regarding Amelogenesis imperfecta except:

(*a*) it can be of hypocalcified,hypomaturation and hypoplastic type

(*b*) taurodontism is sometimes associated with amelogenesis imperfecta

(*c*) jacket crowns can be made for young patients

(*d*) it affects both primary and permanent teeth

(*e*) It is inherited as an autosomal dominant trait only

Answer (*e*).

Amelogenesis imperfecta can be inherited as an autosomal dominant as well as an X-linked type.

28. In Shell Teeth pulp chambers and canals are so enlarged that little more than a shell of enamel and dentin remain. In Dentinogenesis imperfecta the pulp chamber is small or entirely absent, and the pulp canals are small and ribbon like:

(*a*) both the statements are false

(*b*) both the statements are true

(*c*) first statement is true and the second is false

(*d*) first statement is false and the second is true

Answer (*b*).

The question is self-explanatory.

29. Large pulp chambers are characteristic of all of the following conditions except:

(*a*) Shell teeth

(*b*) Dentin dysplasia or dentin aplasia

(*c*) Dentinogenesis imperfecta

(*d*) Taurodontism

Answer (*c*).

In Dentinogenesis imperfecta, the pulp chamber is small or entirely absent and the pulp canals are small and ribbon like.

30. The congenital absence of primary teeth is relatively rare. When a number of the primary teeth fail to develop, other ectodermal deficiencies are usually evident.

(*a*) Both the statements are false.

(*b*) Both the statements are true.

(*c*) First statement is true and the second is false.

(*d*) First statement is false and the second is true.

Answer (*b*).

The answer is self-explanatory. Other deficiencies affecting nails, sweat glands and hair may be seen.

31. Apart from the permanent third molars the most commonly missing permanent tooth is:

(*a*) mandibular second premolars

(*b*) maxillary lateral incisors

(*c*) maxillary second premolars

(*d*) mandibular central incisor

Answer (*a*).

The most commonly missing permanent teeth are the mandibular second premolars, maxillary lateral incisors, and maxillary second premolars. Glenn and Grahnen confirm this order of frequency in their studies.

32. Which of the following is/are true regarding erythroblastosis fetalis?

(*a*) It results from the transplacental passage of maternal antibody active against red blood cell antigens of the infant.

(*b*) Because of persistent jaundice during the neonatal period, the primary teeth may have a characteristic blue green colour or brown colour.

(*c*) The staining of dentin which occurs after birth is due to the perfusion of bilirubin and biliverdin into the dentin.

(*d*) All of the above.

Answer (*d*).

In erythroblastosis fetalis there is massive destruction of the red blood cells by the antigen antibody reaction. All the above-mentioned statements are true regarding erythroblastosis fetalis.

33. A child aged 4 years presents with the following symptoms hypersensitivity to light, passage of red colored urine, blisters on hands and face and purplish brown primary teeth. The most probable diagnosis is:

(*a*) erythroblastosis fetalis

(*b*) porphyria

(*c*) Tetracycline toxicity

(*d*) cystic fibrosis

Answer (*b*).

Children with congenital erythropoietic porphyria have red-colored urine, are hypersensitive to light, and develop sub epidermal bullous lesions when their skin is exposed to sunlight. Their primary teeth are purplish brown as a result of the deposition of porphyrin in the developing structures.

34. Which of the following is/are true regarding tetracycline discoloration?

(*a*) Discoloration is because of chelating properties of tetracycline which forms a tetracycline-calcium orthophosphate complex.

(*b*) Exposure of affected teeth to light results in a color change from yellow to brown (oxidation).

(*c*) The larger the dose of drug relative to body weight the deeper the pigmentation.

(*d*) All the above.

Answer (*d*).

Duration of exposure is less relevant than the total dose relative to body weight. Tetracycline is deposited in the dentin and to a lesser extent in the enamel that is calcifying at that time. Tetracycline when yellow in color fluoresces under ultraviolet light (the fluorescence diminishes when it becomes yellow to brown). If administered during pregnancy crowns of primary teeth show noticeable discoloration. The sensitive period for tetracycline during tooth development is as follows: 4 months in utero to 3 months post partum for maxillary and mandibular incisors, 5months in utero to 9 months post partum for maxillary and mandibular canines, 3 to 5 months post partum to 7th year of life for permanent maxillary, mandibular incisors and canines. Maxillary lateral incisors are an exception because they begin to calcify at 10–12 months post partum. Bleaching with superoxol is a method of managing tetracycline discoloration.

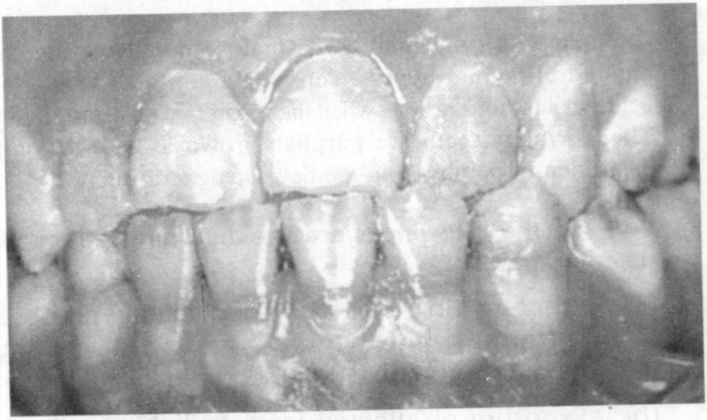

Fig. 24.1 Tetracycline discoloration.

35. Which of the following papillae usually show inflammatory and atrophic changes on the dorsum of the tongue?

(*a*) Fungiform papillae.

(*b*) Foliate papillae.

(*c*) Circumvallate papillae.

(*d*) Filiform papillae.

Answer (*a*).

Inflammatory and atrophic changes occurring on the dorsum of the tongue usually involve the vascularised fungiform papilla.

36. Which of the following papillae are vascularized?

(*a*) Fungiform papillae and circumvallate papillae.

(*b*) Circumvallate papillae and filiform papillae.

(*c*) Filiform papillae and foliate papillae.

(*d*) Foliate papillae and fungiform papillae.

Answer (*a*).

Large circumvallate papillae, 10–15 in number may be found on the posterior border of the dorsum. These papillae have blood supply and they hold numerous taste buds. Fungiform papillae may be distributed over the entire dorsum of the tongue; however, they are present in greater numbers at the tip and towards the lateral margins of the tongue.

37. The papillae associated with taste sensation are:

(*a*) fungiform papillae

(*b*) foliate papillae

(*c*) circumvallate papillae

(*d*) filiform papillae

Answer (*c*).

Foliate papillae are arranged in folds along the lateral margins of the tongue; the taste sensation is associated with these papillae.

38. The most numerous papillae of the tongue are:

(*a*) fungiform papillae

(*b*) foliate papillae

(*c*) circumvallate papillae

(*d*) filiform papillae

Answer (*d*).

The most numerous papillae are the filiform papillae, which are thin and hair like and evenly distributed over the dorsal surface. The filiform papillae are without a vascular core and their continuous growth is slight.

39. All of the following conditions are associated with Macroglossia except:

(*a*) cretinism

(*b*) Down syndrome

(*c*) angio neurotic edema

(*d*) ectodermal dysplasia

Answer (*d*).

Macroglossia refers to a larger than normal size of the tongue. This can be congenital or acquired. Congenital macroglossia caused by an overdevelopment of the lingual musculature or vascular tissues becomes increasingly apparent as the child develops.

40. Which of the following patients can have fissured tongue?

(*a*) Down syndrome

(*b*) Cretinism

(*c*) Vit B complex deficiency

(*d*) Any of the above

Answer (*d*).

The answer is self-explanatory.

41. Which of the following pairs regarding the papillary distribution is incorrect?

(*a*) Circumvallate papillae-posterior border of the dorsum.

(*b*) Fungiform papillae-tips and lateral borders predominantly (also entire dorsum).

(*c*) Filiform papillae-even distribution over the dorsum.

(*d*) Foliate papillae-middle of the tongue.

Answer (*d*).

Refer to the explanations of Q. Nos. 36, 37 and 38.

42. Scarlet fever is associated with:

(*a*) strawberry tongue

(*b*) coated tongue

(*c*) fissured tongue

(*d*) black hairy tongue

Answer (*a*).

An enlargement of the fungiform papillae extending above the level of the white desquamating filiform papillae gives the appearance of an unripe strawberry. This condition has been observed in cases of scarlet fever and Kawasaki disease in young children.

43. Strawberry tongue is because of:

(*a*) enlargement of filiform papillae

(*b*) enlargement of fungiform papillae

(*c*) enlargement of foliate papillae

(*d*) enlargement of circumvallate papillae

Answer (*b*).

Refer to the explanation of Q. No. 42.

44. Which of the following tongue anomaly is associated with Candida albicans?

(*a*) Median rhomboid glossitis.

(*b*) Black hairy tongue.

(*c*) Strawberry tongue.

(*d*) Benign migratory glossitis.

Answer (*a*).

Median rhomboid glossitis is an oval, rhomboid, or diamond shaped reddish patch on the dorsal surface of the tongue immediately anterior to the circumvallate papillae.

45. Which of the following tongue anomaly is associated with oral and systemic intake of antibiotics?

(*a*) Median rhomboid glossitis.

(*b*) Black hairy tongue.

(*c*) Strawberry tongue.

(*d*) Benign migratory glossitis.

Answer (*b*).

Black hairy tongue is rarely seen in children but occurs in young adults and has been related to the oral and systemic intake of antibiotics, smoking, and excessive ingestion of dark drinks such as coffee and tea. Accumulations of keratin on the filiform papillae in the middle third of the tongue become elongated into hair like processes, sometimes as long as 2.5 cm (1 inch).

46. Which of the following can cause midline diastema?

(*a*) Oral habits.

(*b*) Supernumerary tooth.

(*c*) Macroglossia.

(*d*) Peg lateral and congenital absence of permanent lateral incisors.

(*e*) Abnormal labial frenum.

(*f*) Any of the above.

Answer (*f*).

The answer is self-explanatory.

47. The labial frenum is composed of two layers of epithelium enclosing a loose vascular connective tissue. Muscle fibers if present are derived from the zygomaticus major muscle.

(*a*) Both the statements are false.

(*b*) Both the statements are true.

(*c*) First statement is true and the second is false.

(*d*) First statement is false and the second is true.

Answer (*c*).

Muscle fibers for the labial frenum are derived from the Orbicularis oris muscle.

48. An abnormal labial frenum can cause

(*a*) interference with tooth brushing

(*b*) stripping of tissue from neck of tooth

(*c*) accumulation of food particles which leads to pocket formation

(*d*) interference with speech

(*e*) any of the above

Answer (*e*).

The answer is self-explanatory.

Chapter 25

Child Abuse and Neglect

1. The first documented and reported case of child abuse occurred in:

(*a*) 1874 (*b*) 1974

(*c*) 1894 (*d*) 1924

Answer (*a*).

The first documented and reported case of child abuse occurred in 1874. A child named Mary Ellen was discovered chained to her bedpost. She was beaten regularly and was found to be severely malnourished. A New York City Church group reported the situation to the police.

2. The term battered-child syndrome was coined by (in 1962):

(*a*) Caffey (*b*) Mary Ellen

(*c*) Henry Kempe (*d*) Needleman

Answer (*c*).

Henry Kempe coined the term battered-child syndrome in his milestone article in 1962. Caffey and Silverman reported cases of child abuse in their article. Mary Ellen is the name of the first documented child who was reported to be abused. Needleman reported cases of child abuse with orofacial trauma.

3. Battered child syndrome should be considered in any child exhibiting evidence of:

(*a*) fractures of any long bone

(*b*) subdural hematomas

(*c*) failure to thrive, soft tissue swelling or skin bruising

(*d*) any of the above

Answer (*d*).

According to Henry Kempe battered child syndrome should be considered in any child exhibiting evidence of fractures of any long bone, subdural hematoma, failure to thrive, soft tissue swelling and skin bruising.

4. Which one of the following is/are a form of child abuse and neglect?

(*a*) Munchausen syndrome by proxy

(*b*) Sexual abuse or exploitation

(*c*) Intentional drugging or poisoning

(*d*) All of the above

Answer (*d*).

All the above mentioned conditions are different forms of child abuse and neglect. Munchausen syndrome by proxy is a form of fabricated illness by the parents. Sexual abuse is a form of child abuse where an adult sexually exploits the child. Intentional drugging or poisoning is a form of child abuse where the child is drugged or poisoned by the caretaker.

5. All of the following is / are true regarding physical abuse except:

(*a*) otherwise known as accidental trauma

(*b*) defined as injuries inflicted on a person under 18 years of age by a caretaker

(*c*) graded from mild, to moderate and severe forms of abuse

(*d*) usually recognized by the pattern of injury or its inconsistency with the history related

Answer (*a*).

Physical abuse is defined as non-accidental trauma. The injuries in physical abuse are graded from mild (a few bruises, welts, or scratches) to moderate (numerous bruises, minor burns, or a single fracture) to severe (large burns, CNS injury, abdominal injury, multiple fractures, or other life threatening injuries). A careful history by an alert clinician will reveal inconsistency in the history from the parent and the child. Also the type and severity of the injuries may not coincide with the history.

6. All of the following are true regarding failure to thrive except:

(*a*) a child who is overweight

(*b*) when a child fails to grow and develop because of insufficient caloric intake

(*c*) usually under 2 years of age

(*d*) can be shown to thrive once they are removed from the home and placed on unlimited feedings of a normal diet for their age

Answer (*a*).

In failure to thrive the child is underweight and malnourished.

7. One of the following statements regarding Munchausen syndrome by proxy is false:

(*a*) children who are victims of parentally fabricated or induced illnesses

(*b*) involvement of children who are too young (under 6 years of age) to be aware of or able to tell others about this deception

(*c*) fabricated illnesses which may lead to unnecessary medical treatment

(*d*) bleeding from various sites, recurrent sepsis from injecting contaminated fluids, chronic diarrhea from laxatives, fevers or skin rashes as their signs and symptoms

(*e*) Fractures of long bones, sub-dural hematomas and soft tissue swellings or skin bruising are characteristic clinical features

Answer (*e*).

Munchausen syndrome by proxy is a malignant disorder of parenting in which the caretaker (usually the mother) relates a factitious history, produces false signs and symptoms and fabricates illnesses in the child. It results in extensive medical evaluations, testing and often-prolonged hospitalizations. Choice "e" has characteristic features of battered-child syndrome.

8. All of the following is/are true regarding Health care neglect except:

(*a*) when a parent or caretaker ignores the treatment recommendations of a health professional for the management of a treatable illness that a child has and is becoming worse is health care neglect

(*b*) dental neglect is a specific type of health care neglect

(*c*) AAPD defines dental neglect as the failure by a parent or a guardian to seek treatment for visually untreated caries, oral infection and or oral pain or failure of the parent or guardian to follow through with treatment once informed that the above conditions exists

(*d*) Continual scapegoat and rejection of a child by parents, caretakers or teachers

Answer (*d*).

Continual scapegoat and rejection of a child by parents, caretakers or teachers is a type of emotional abuse.

9. Match the following:

S. No.	*Type of abuse*	*S. No.*	*Description*
1.	Safety neglect	A	Continual scapegoat and rejection of a child by parents, caretakers or teachers
2.	Emotional abuse	B	Includes inadequate nurturance or affection, i.e. lack of "mothering", knowingly "permitted" maladaptive behaviour such as delinquency or substance abuse
3.	Emotional neglect	C	Failure to care for a child according to accepted or appropriate standards
4.	Physical neglect	D	When a parent or caretaker knowingly permits chronic truancy, intentionally keeps the child home, or fails to enroll the child in school
5.	Educational abuse	E	Gross lack of direct or indirect supervision of a child which results in an injury

(*a*) 1-E, 2-A, 3-B, 4-C, 5-D
(*b*) 1-D, 2-E, 3-A, 4-B, 5-C
(*c*) 1-B, 2-C, 3-D, 4-E, 5-A
(*d*) 1-A, 2-B, 3-C, 4-D, 5-E

Answer (*a*).

The above mentioned table describes or defines safety neglect, emotional abuse, emotional neglect, physical neglect and educational abuse.

10. All of the following statements regarding an abused child are true except:

(*a*) trauma to the head and associated areas occurs in approximately 50% of the cases of physical abuse to children

(*b*) soft tissue injuries (most frequently bruises) are the most common injuries sustained by the head and face and are the single-most common injury sustained in child abuse

(*c*) injury to the upper lip and maxillary labial frenum may be a characteristic lesion in the severely abused young child

(*d*) the youngest children (infancy to two years) tend to be sexually abused most often

Answer (*d*).

Usually the youngest children (infancy to two years) tend to be neglected most often and sexually or emotionally abused least often. On the other hand, older children (12–17 years) are the least neglected but the most sexually and emotionally abused.

11. Most difficult form of child maltreatment to identify and treat is:

(*a*) sexual abuse

(*b*) physical abuse

(*c*) emotional abuse

(*d*) munchausen syndrome by proxy

Answer (*d*).

Munchausen syndrome by proxy is a malignant disorder of parenting in which the parents (usually mother) relates a fictitious history, produces false signs or symptoms, and fabricates illnesses in the child that result in extensive medical evaluations, testing and often prolonged hospitalizations. Because health care providers are often dependent on the parental history of the child's illness it takes sometime for the practitioner to realize the inconsistencies and possibly fabricated or exaggerated nature of the complaints. Hence, it is very difficult to identify and treat Munchausen syndrome by proxy. The other names of this condition are factitious disorder by proxy and pediatric condition falsification.

12. The Child Abuse Prevention and Treatment Act was signed into law in United States in:

(*a*) 1974 (*b*) 1932

(*c*) 1986 (*d*) 1956

Answer (*a*).

In 1974, the Child Abuse Prevention and Treatment Act was signed into law. It established for the first time within the federal government a national center on Child Abuse and Neglect.

13. Which of the following is an evidence for sexual abuse?

(*a*) Tearing, bruising, or specific inflammation of the mouth, anus, or genitals.

(*b*) Venereal disease of the mouth, eyes, anus or genitals in a child under 15.

(*c*) Pregnancy and the girl is very evasive in naming her partner.

(*d*) Any of the above.

Answer (*d*).

The answer is self-explanatory.

14. A child aged 4 years reports with the following findings: undernourished, small for age, symptoms of malnutrition with dirty clothes. This is classified as:

(*a*) physical neglect (*b*) emotional abuse

(*c*) emotional neglect (*d*) physical abuse

Answer (*a*).

Refer the explanation of Q. No. 9.

15. Which of the following characterizes an abuser?

(*a*) Abuser may demonstrate psychotic behavior.

(*b*) Abuser may view the child as different or bad.

(*c*) When the abuser is confronted with allegations of abuse, he or she makes no attempt to explain the injuries.

(*d*) Any of the above.

Answer (*d*).

The answer is self-explanatory. Child abuse is seldom the result of any single factor. Usually it is due to a combination of emotional and environmental stresses, a predisposition towards maltreatment, a personality type, an occasion when for some reason the child happens to trigger the parent's contempt or resentment.

Chapter 26

Cleft Lip, Palate Management and Speech Therapy

1. The most frequently used classification of cleft lip was given by:

(*a*) Veau

(*b*) Kernahan and Starke

(*c*) classification of Cleft Palate Association

(*d*) classification of American Association of Cleft Lip and Palate

Answer (*a*).

Veau's classification of cleft lip is as follows:

Class I – Unilateral notching of vermilion not extending to the lip.

Class II – Unilateral notching of vermilion border with cleft extending into the lip but not including the floor of the nose.

Class III – Unilateral clefting of the vermilion border of the lip extending into the floor of the nose.

Class IV – Any bilateral clefting of the lip whether it is incomplete notching or complete clefting.

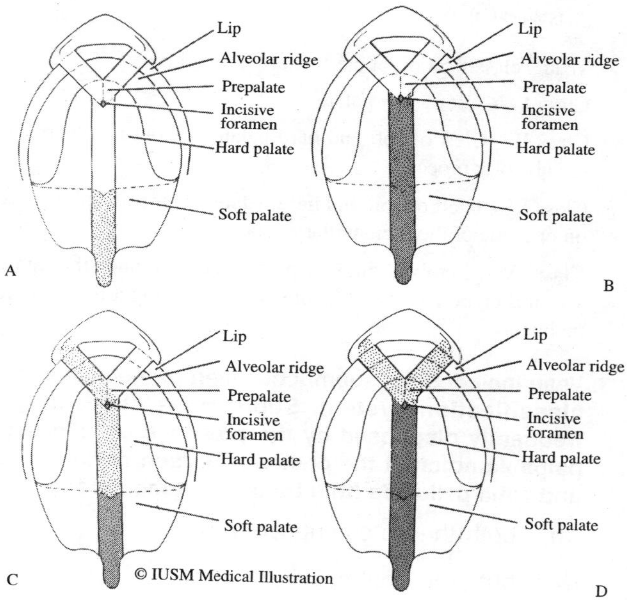

Fig. 26.1 Veau's classification of cleft lip and palate.

2. Which of the following regarding Veau's classification of cleft palate is incorrect?

(*a*) Class I – Cleft of soft palate.

(*b*) Class II – Cleft of soft and hard palate with alveolar process.

(*c*) Class III – Cleft of soft and hard palate and alveolar process on one side of premaxillary area.

(*d*) Class IV – Involves soft palate, continues through alveolus on both sides of premaxilla leaving it free and often mobile.

Answer (b).

Veau's classification of cleft palate is as follows:

Class I – Cleft of soft palate

Class II – Cleft of soft and hard palate without involvement of the alveolar process

Class III – Cleft of soft and hard palate and the alveolar process on one side of the premaxillary area

Class IV – Involves the soft palate and continues through the alveolus on both sides of the premaxilla, leaving it free and often mobile

3. Veau included the submucous cleft of the palate in his classification system. Submucous clefts may be frequently diagnosed by the presence of bifid uvula, palpable notch at the posterior portion of hard palate and zona pellucida (thin translucent membrane):

(*a*) both the statements are false

(*b*) both the statements are true

(*c*) first statement is true and the second is false

(*d*) first statement is false and the second is true

Answer (d).

Veau did not include submucous cleft of the palate in his classification system.

Refer to the explanation of Q. No. 2.

4. Which of the following anomalies are associated with cleft lip and palate?

(*a*) Natal teeth and neonatal teeth.

(*b*) Congenitally missing teeth.

(*c*) Increase in presence of supernumerary teeth.

(*d*) Any of the above.

Answer (*d*).

All of the above mentioned features are associated with cleft lip and palate.

Natal teeth (teeth found at birth) and neonatal teeth (teeth that erupt within first 30 days after birth) are usually maxillary central incisors observed in patients with a complete unilateral or bilateral cleft palate. There is high incidence of congenitally missing teeth especially the primary or permanent lateral incisors (adjacent to the cleft) and premolars. Supernumerary teeth are often seen in those with complete unilateral or bilateral clefts.

5. With a complete cleft of the palate and alveolus there is no longer a contiguous maxillary arch. External forces applied to muscles of mastication or the contraction of scar tissue subsequent to surgical repair of cleft palate can result in medial collapse of posterior segments causing posterior crossbite.

(*a*) Both the statements are false.

(*b*) Both the statements are true.

(*c*) First statement is true and the second is false.

(*d*) First statement is false and the second is true.

Answer (*b*).

The answer is self-explanatory.

6. The initial surgical closure of cleft lip is done at:

(*a*) 6 months

(*b*) 3 months

(*c*) 1 year and 6 months

(*d*) 2 years

Answer (b).

Surgical closure of cleft lip is usually accomplished at 10 weeks of age (3 months).

7. The rule of tens used in determining optimal timing of surgical lip closure considers which of the following:

(*a*) age (*b*) weight

(*c*) hemoglobin (*d*) all of the above

Answer (d).

Rule of Tens says that the child should be 10 months of age, weighing 10 pounds and having 10 gm of hemoglobin to undergo any surgical procedure.

8. Which of the following statements regarding palatoplasty is/are true?

(*a*) Palatoplasty (surgical closure of palate) is usually accomplished between 12 months and 2 years of age.

(*b*) The primary purpose of palatal closure by 2 years of age is to facilitate the acquisition of normal speech.

(*c*) The procedure may also improve hearing and swallowing by aligning the cleft palatal musculature.

(*d*) All of the above.

Answer (d).

The answer is self-explanatory.

9. Lefort I maxillary advancement is not technically feasible until the patient has a full complement of

permanent dentition. The horizontal cuts to free the maxilla must necessarily be made above the apices of permanent dentition; hence unerupted cuspids or bicuspids would make the procedure impractical.

(*a*) Both the statements are false.

(*b*) Both the statements are true.

(*c*) First statement is true and the second is false.

(*d*) First statement is false and the second is true.

Answer (*b*).

The answer is self-explanatory.

10. Speech may be observed as the ordered utterance of language. It is controlled by four basic processes called respiration, phonation, resonance and articulation.

(*a*) Both the statements are false.

(*b*) Both the statements are true.

(*c*) First statement is true and the second is false.

(*d*) First statement is false and the second is true.

Answer (*b*).

The answer is self-explanatory.

11. All of the following statements regarding speech sounds are true except:

(*a*) the two major categories of speech sounds in the English language are vowels and consonants

(*b*) consonants are the first speech sounds to be fully mastered

(*c*) vowels are produced with minimal constriction of vocal tract (by open vocal tract) (*d*) consonants are produced by constriction or obstruction of vocal tract (closed vocal tract)

Answer (*b*).

Vowels are the first speech sounds to be fully mastered. Most children articulate vowels by 3–31/2 years. Consonant sounds require more time to master. Consonant sound maturation remains incomplete even at 8 years.

12. Impairment of velo-pharyngeal motion has been demonstrated in which of the following conditions:

(*a*) cleft palate

(*b*) poliomyelitis

(*c*) myasthenia gravis

(*d*) muscular dystrophy

(*e*) all of the above

Answer (*e*).

All of the above mentioned conditions affect the muscular function. Hence impairment of velopharyngeal motion is seen in all the above mentioned conditions.

13. Stuttering typically begins in childhood between 2.5–4 years of age. Stuttering is characterized by breakdowns (repetitions, prolongations and hesitations) in the rhythm or fluency of speech.

(*a*) Both the statements are false.

(*b*) Both the statements are true.

(*c*) First statement is true and the second is false.

(*d*) First statement is false and the second is true.

Answer (*b*).

The answer is self-explanatory.

14. Cleft lip occurs due to non-union of:

(*a*) maxillary and frontonasal processes

(*b*) maxillary and mandibular process

(*c*) maxillary process and palatine process

(*d*) medial nasal process and maxillary process

Answer (*d*).

The answer is self-explanatory.